Confessions of a Body Builder

Rejuvenating the Body with Spirulina, Chlorella, Raw Foods and Ionized Water

by

Bob McCauley

This book is dedicated to my father, Dr. Robert McCauley, Sr., my mother, sister and two sons Daniel and Phillip. With their love, support, patience (and quiet) I was able to complete this book.

I would also like to thank Mr. Minsok Kim for his support of the Watershed and this project and to Jim Hatch for being my best customer and a great friend. And to all on The Watershed Wellness Center Team, past, present and future.

August 17, 2000

2nd Edition, June 2003
3rd Edition, May 2005

This book is not intended in any way to serve as a replacement for professional medical advice. Rather, it is meant to demonstrate that aging can be slowed and even reversed and that great health is achieved when the most fundamental nutritional needs of the human body are met. Always consult a doctor or another medical professional when you have an illness or disease of any kind.

Edited by: Nathan T. Anderson (2nd Edition)

Spartan Enterprises, Inc.
Robert F. McCauley, Jr.
The Watershed Wellness Center
www.ionizedwater.com

Introduction

I am not a body builder in the sense one usually thinks of a body builder. I do not sit in a gym with other muscular men and women and pump iron. While I do exercise vigorously everyday, the *body building* I refer to in the title of this book, and on the following pages, has to do with rejuvenating our bodies at the cellular level through the use of *Nutrients* and *Ionized Water*. What is accomplished by this is nothing short of *slowing, if not reversing, the aging process*. Much to my amazement, it can be done!

I am not a doctor, certified nutritionist or trained medical professional of any kind. Perhaps my distance from these professions has given me a perspective that has not been clouded by the insistence of some that until something has been studied in double-blind tests and included in a standardized medical textbook, it simply can't be true. Keep in mind that if money can't be made from it, it won't be studied.

Take, for instance, the role of alkalinity in human health. I am not alone in the belief that keeping the body alkaline and balanced is key to fighting disease of any kind. *Disease loves an acid environment*. However, the medical establishment has yet to accept this basic principle. Instead, it looks puzzled and suggests vaguely that environmental, genetic or some other unknown factors must be the culprit when asked why cancer and heart disease rates continue at historically high levels. The importance of alkalinity in the body and its relationship to human health will be discussed later in this book, but suffice to say that if you create an acidic environment in your body through poor diet, you have opened yourself up to a host of diseases and ailments, most of which can be held in check if you simply keep your body's pH properly balanced.

There is plenty of hard scientific evidence that fresh fruit and vegetables are quite healthy, build the body and prevent disease, but it is barely mentioned by the medical community beyond an asterisk because things that prevent disease are not big money makers.

My interest in healthy eating began over 20 years ago. I stumbled onto vegetarianism almost by accident and found I felt better after removing meat from my diet. I had more energy and mental alertness. I was raised on junk food and the difference was even more dramatic once I removed most of the processed foods from my diet. I stopped consuming soft drinks, which is one of the most profoundly beneficial health decisions anyone can ever make. I was careful to make sure the four vegetarian protein sources were in my diet: beans & legumes, dairy products, seeds & nuts and grains (wheat, rye, oats, etc.).

Supplementing them with superior whole foods such as *Spirulina & Chlorella* came nearly 17 years later. They are the perfect health compliment to the human body because they contain the exact nutrients the body needs. Literally nothing on earth compares with their power and nutraceutical prowess. However, the most important element the body must have is WATER and the best water to drink is **Ionized Water**.

We will touch on all these subjects in the coming pages, including the Three Principles of Great Health. We will focus on what we put in the body now, what we ought not to put in the body and what we must put in the body if we expect to truly rejuvenate it. The human body regenerates and replaces all its cells approximately every seven years. *From which foods are you getting the nutrients that your body's cells must have in order stay healthy and young?* If the answer is soft drinks, cooked foods, fast foods, junk and otherwise processed foods, don't wonder why you ache here and there and are looking a little bit older every other glance in the mirror. You are aging and the food you are eating is accelerating it. But you can slow it down, even reverse it.

I would also like to make a promise not to become too technical in explaining any of the foods and ideas promoted in this book. It's the easiest way to lose the reader and you don't need to know how a fuel injector works to drive a car. I will explain basic principles of how *Spirulina* and *Chlorella*, raw foods and *Ionized Water* can enhance our health and our lives, but I will not delve into the physical, chemical or biological detail of how and why it works. That book I will leave to someone else to write, and to those who want to read it.

PART ONE

Chapter 1

"The preservation of health is a duty. Few seem conscious that there is such a thing as physical morality." -- Herbert Spencer

Water: The Beginning of Life

Water is the universal solvent. Without it, life could not exist. It assures the wheel of life continues: birth, death and renewal. It is the most common substance found on Earth. Water covers 80% of our planet, but only 3% is fresh water, most of it stored frozen in glaciers.

Algae, the first food on the planet billions of years ago, could not exist till there was water. Bacteria, the most primordial life form, cannot exist without water. The human body is 69% water, the human brain 85% water, human bones 25% water and human blood 83% water.

Water is the body's most vital need, yet it is entirely ignored by scores of people who couldn't begin to tell you when they last drank a glass of water. When the sun is high and hot, they reach for a soft drink to quench their thirst and end up dramatically dehydrating themselves and leaching out vital electrolytes, sometimes to dangerous levels. The human body can only survive three days without water. The average person loses nearly 2.5 liters of water every day due to perspiration, respiration, urination and defecation. This must be replaced on a continuous basis. Failure to do so results in an imbalance of vital fluids as well as a host of other bodily disparities, biases and deterioration.

"The role of water itself in the body of living species, mankind included, has not changed since the first creation of life from salt water and its subsequent adaptation to fresh water." [1]

The human body craves water. It is our body's solvent, something akin to what grease is to a machine. It lubricates our joints and organs. Water assists our muscles, heart, tissue, every cell and organ of the body to function optimally. It is our greatest cleanser and detoxifier, carrying away poisons and toxins of all kinds. It prevents premature aging of the skin and internal body tissue. It is the primary ingredient in our blood. When the optimal blood volume is reached through adequate intake of water, nutrients we consume are properly transported to every part of the body.

The brain uses 80% of the water we drink. Consuming too much alcohol gives people a headache the following morning because it drastically dehydrates the fluids around the brain, sometimes to the point that the brain itself is resting against the skull.

Not drinking enough water will cause the body to actually retain water! Many people, even doctors, recommend that people stop drinking water to curb its retention, but no prescription could be worse. Water becomes stored in extra-cellular areas, outside the cells, which manifests itself as swollen legs, hands and feet. Diuretics offer temporary relief at best, but as the water is driven out of these areas, essential minerals are lost with it. The body reacts by replacing the lost water at its first opportunity and the condition of bloating soon returns. The only way to rid the body of retained water is to drink plenty of water. Sometimes water retention is caused by excess sodium (salt). The body retains water in order to dilute the high sodium concentration in the body. The only way to rid the body of the excess sodium is to force it out through the kidneys by drinking more water.

Water regulates our body's optimal weight by helping it to properly digest the food we eat, and to eliminate the waste. Drinking adequate amounts of water naturally suppresses the appetite while helping to decrease fat deposits by metabolizing them. Without enough water, the food we eat is not properly hydrated, therefore it does not pass through the body as quickly nor have its nutrients absorbed as readily by the body during the digestive process. This condition can lead to constipation, which can in turn lead to hemorrhoids. A slow moving digestive system is also associated with some types of cancer.

"Chronic and persistently increasing dehydration is the root cause of almost all currently encountered major disease of the human body." [2] Dehydration can seriously impair kidney function. The kidneys produce urine that carries away toxins from the body. If this condition becomes chronic, the body will retain water as a natural defense against dehydration, which can cause bloating and other maladies.

Any weight-loss diet should be accompanied by consuming large amounts of water. In fact, weight loss cannot be accomplished in a healthful way if the body is not sufficiently hydrated. If water is not present in the body, stored fat cells cannot be properly metabolized, or used up as fuel by the body. Water provides tone to the muscles and prevents wrinkled, sagging skin that often appears after weight loss.

Drinking cold water can lead to weight loss because it causes the body to raise its metabolism in order to produce heat and maintain an internal body temperature of 98.6° F. This process is known as *thermogenesis.* It is this state of increased metabolism, which causes the body to expend energy and burn fat.

"High blood pressure, hypertension, is a result of an adaptive process to a gross body water deficiency." [3]

Years of reaching for something to drink other than water has unfortunately trained many people not to drink water when they most need it. When the body is receiving enough water, our natural thirst urge returns. People who rarely drink enough water have suppressed the urge of thirst to the point that they no longer realize their body is crying out every moment of every day for more water.

"Chronic cellular dehydration painfully and prematurely kills. Its initial outward manifestations have until now been labeled as diseases of unknown origin." [4] *In his book,* Your Body's Many Cries For Water, F. Batmanghelidj contends that many diseases can be traced to dehydration at a cellular level where the body's cells are only hydrated from 70% - 90% of their total requirements, which leaves them in a perpetually weakened and defensive posture. Given this kind of chronically dehydrated state, the cell can never function as it was designed to.

Almost all liquids other than water itself do not actually provide the body with much water at all. The reason is because it takes water for the body to process liquids such as juice, milk, coffee, tea, caffienated drinks, alcohol and especially carbonated soft drinks, *which significantly dehydrate the body.*

"In advanced societies, thinking that tea, coffee, alcohol and manufactured beverages are desirable substitutes for the purely natural needs of the daily "stressed" body is an elementary but

catastrophic mistake. It is true that these beverages contain water, but what else they contain are dehydrating agents." [5]

We do not educate our children to drink water, but rather accustom them to consume soft drinks, processed juices, milk and ultra-sweet juice drinks. Water is not typically a part of a child's routine in any way. For instance, children are not taught to drink a large glass of water just after waking in the morning. However, you will find that if you put a water cooler in your house, children will go for the water and leave the soft drinks and other beverages in the fridge. This is because the human body naturally, as well as subconsciously, tells us which substances it needs, which substances are good for it and what we should be drinking.

"The most toxic commercial beverages that people consume (i.e. cola beverages and other soft drinks) are made from purified water. Studies have consistently shown that heavy consumers of soft drinks (with or without sugar) spill huge amounts of calcium, magnesium and other trace minerals into the urine. The more mineral loss, the greater the risk for osteoporosis, osteoarthritis, hypothyroidism, coronary artery disease, high blood pressure and a long list of degenerative diseases generally associated with premature aging." [6]

The medical establishment is not trained to prescribe water as a treatment or *preventive health* measure against disease. There is little, if any, mention of water in today's medical textbooks, yet nothing is more vital to human health. This is occurring in part because the medical establishment does not routinely suggest *preventative health* measures that help forestall disease to begin with. *"Medical professionals of today do not understand the vital roles of water in the human body. Medications are palliatives. They are not designed to cure the degenerative diseases of the human body."* [7]

I want to state for the record that I have nothing against doctors or the medical establishment. However, in many cases they are arrogantly close-minded to some of the most obvious causes and cures of human disease.

"Physicians think they are doing something for you by labeling what you have as a disease." [8] For instance, most doctors will not consider *Ionized Water* to be of any medical benefit, regardless of what it reportedly does for the body. They will not consider the possibility

that magnets are helpful in fighting pain and healing injuries. They scoff at most herbs and whole food nutraceuticals such as *Spirulina* and *Chlorella.* At best, they suggest they may have some limited benefit for some people, but they never go so far as to actually prescribe them for ailments.

There is a right time and a wrong time to drink water. Any time is the right time except 30 minutes before a meal, during a meal and at least 30 minutes after a meal. Drinking any liquid during mealtime is highly inadvisable because it impedes the digestive process. *(See Great Digestion)*

Drinking any liquids during mealtime, including water, serves only to dilute digestion and leave food to rot in the gut instead of being properly digested. It is true that water is used abundantly in the digestive process, but it needs to be there well before the food is eaten. Not drinking any liquids just before, during and after a meal may take a little getting use to, but the benefits of great digestion, not artificially induced by some drug, are well worth it.

Always drink water before you are thirsty. By doing this, you will always remain hydrated. Disease has a tougher time getting a foothold in the body because when it is well hydrated its organs, tissue and cells will have their best opportunity to fight disease. Athletic performance is also at its peak when the body is well hydrated and hampered when it is not.

A standard rule of thumb for how much water we should drink is half our body weight in ounces daily to provide the body with its MINIMUM water requirements. For instance, if a person weighs 200 lbs., they should drink 100 ounces of water per day minimum. Doubling or tripling that intake wouldn't hurt a bit.

Top Ten Reasons We Need To Drink Water

1. Water is the substance of life. **Life cannot exist without water.** We must constantly add fresh water to the body in order to keep it properly hydrated. We can only survive three days without water. It is imperative we always remain sufficiently hydrated.

2. The body is comprised of 69% water. This ratio must be maintained for optimal health. **No element we put in our body is more important than water.**

3. **It is difficult for the body to get water from any source other than water itself.** Soft drinks and alcohol steal tremendous amounts of water from the body. Even other beverages such as coffee, milk and juice require water from the body to be processed.
4. **Water plays a vital role in nearly every bodily function.**
5. Water is essential for proper digestion, nutrient absorption, chemical and enzyme reactions.
6. Water is essential for proper circulation in the body.
7. Water helps remove toxins from the body, in particular from the digestive track.
8. Water regulates the body's cooling system.
9. **Consistent failure to drink enough water will lead to *Chronic Cellular Dehydration.*** This is a condition where the body's cells are never quite hydrated to their capacity so they are constantly in a weakened state, vulnerable to attack from disease. It weakens the body's overall immune system and leads to chemical, hormonal nutritional and pH imbalances that can lead to a host of diseases.
10. Dehydration can occur at any time of the year, not only during the summer months when it is hot. The dryness that occurs during winter months can dehydrate the body even quicker than when it is hot. Many victims of various diseases such as cholera die primarily from dehydration, not the disease itself.

Water is by far the most important substance we consume. Drink half your weight in ounces of water daily is the *rule that should rule you.* **Water is vital to every cell in the body, every biological process and every vital component of human health.**

The quality of water we drink is also of paramount importance. Below is a brief overview of available waters.

Which Water to Drink

My family has been involved in water technology in one capacity or another for over 50 years. We know water, good, bad and otherwise. My father, Robert F. McCauley, Sr., was a renown water expert. He received a doctorate from the Massachusetts Institute of Technology, taught Environmental Engineering at Michigan State University for 25 years then ran an engineering company for 17 years. We have been in the bottled water business since the early 1990's.

Although certain areas are high in iron, which negatively effects its taste, Michigan has exceptional water in great abundance. I am specifically referring to the ground water in Michigan, not the Great Lakes. Michigan's ground water is naturally filtered through several geologic strata before reaching its sandstone acquifer where it is drawn. It takes rain water about 50 years to filter through layers of gravel, clay, sand, silt and limestone before it reaches the white sandstone acquifer 200-400 feet below. Clay offers the perfect filtration for natural and artificial pollutants of any kind. Essentially, nothing gets through clay except water itself.

Certainly, not all water is as clean and good tasting as Michigan's. However, there are several options in choosing a good drinking water.

Bottled Water

There are hundreds of bottled waters on the market. The vast majority of US bottled waters are good quality. The standards set by the EPA (Environmental Protection Agency) and FDA (Food and Drug Administration) are extremely strict and not easy to circumvent. FDA standards require filtration and ozonation of all bottled water with accurate labeling that declares the exact source of the water. These guidelines are strict and ensure that US bottled water is some of the best in the world.

Frankly, expensive foreign brands are not worth the money. Shipping water great distances is quite costly. To take something as common as good drinking water and transform it into gold because it's been shipped half way around the world is a ridiculous proposition.

Purified Water

(Distilled or Reverse Osmosis)

Do not drink purified water. It is water that has had all the minerals removed from so it is literally pure H_2O. Because of its purity, it absorbs carbon dioxide out of the air, which makes it acidic and even more aggressive at dissolving alkaline substances it comes in contact with. It usually contains little or no dissolved oxygen and therefore is considered *dead water*, which is another reason why it should not be consumed. Purified water leaches minerals from the body, turning the body more acidic. It goes into the body pure, but does not come out pure.

"The longer one drinks purified water, the more likely the development of mineral deficiencies and an acid state. Disease and early death is more likely to be seen with the long term drinking of purified water." [9]

Since it is pure H_2O, it naturally seeks to balance or mollify its extremely pure condition with an alkaline buffer. What is immediately available are the alkaline minerals of the body, thus they are absorbed by the pure water and carried away as it leaves the body. While pure water carries away toxins, it will also take with it vital minerals and other elements needed by the body.

Purified water became a popular fad in the 1970's and remains so to this day with some doctors in the health food, and alternative medicine industries. People who regularly drink purified water often have chronic digestive problems such as gas and diarrhea. Fasting with purified water can be extremely dangerous since it quickly depletes the body of its vital minerals. One person reported his hair turned gray within two weeks of fasting with purified water because it so quickly depleted the copper from his body.

Proponents of drinking purified water suggest first that the minerals in non-purified water will collect in the veins over time and become like cement, which is an absurd and entirely unsupported notion. There is absolutely no evidence to suggest this would happen. Elderly people who have consumed water with a high mineral content all their lives have shown no indication of this condition in their veins whatsoever.

Proponents of purified water will also claim that the amount of minerals in water are small, about what is found in a slice of orange compared to an eight ounce glass of water. This misses the point entirely. The reason mineral water is better to drink is because the minerals provide a crucial buffer which prevents minerals from being leached from the body. If the water you drink already has minerals, physics dictates that it will not try to leach more into it because it is already balanced.

Ironically, FDA labeling regulations state that only water purified by reverse osmosis or distillation can be labeled *Drinking Water*. Leave it to regulators to confuse the public on this issue, but it is crucial. Don't consume anything labeled *Drinking Water* because it will leach minerals from your body.

Spring Water

This is the most common type of bottled water found on the market. Whether it is always true or not, spring water is synonymous with good tasting water. Spring water is ground water that has been naturally pushed to the surface, usually from deep within the earth. However, this means the water has been exposed to surface ground water and air pollution. For this reason, the FDA requires that spring water be filtered below one micron before being ozonated. Most spring water found on the market is good quality as long as the TDS (*Total Dissolved Solids* or amount of minerals in the water) is above 50 ppm (parts per million).

Mineral & Artesian Water

Mineral water must contain a TDS of at least 375 ppm of minerals for it to be labeled a mineral water. Some countries demand higher TDS levels than that. Mineral water is often some of the best tasting water until is reaches a TDS over 550 ppm.

Artesian water is usually considered high quality water; however, this depends geographically on where the source is. Artesian water is well water typically drawn from a deep source below 150' and often falls into the same category as mineral water because it tends to be high in mineral content. Technically, artesian water must be drawn from a static water level that is higher than the actual acquifer. Therefore, it must have enough pressure to be forced upward through the confining bed to a level higher than the acquifer. For instance, if the acquifer is 200' down, the water must be drawn at a depth of 150' or higher. Artesian water does not have to flow from the well-head for the well to be considered artesian. Such a well that is constantly flowing is called a *flowing artesian well*. Unlike spring water, artesian water has not been exposed to surface ground water and air pollution because it is draw from a well, which is a distinct advantage.

Municipal Water

(*Tap Water* or *City Water*)

Although there are definitely problems in some areas, most municipal tap water in the US is fit to drink except for the fact that they all contain chlorine, which is added to kill bacteria in the water.

Unfortunately, chlorine is a proven carcinogen and quite dangerous, even if consumed in very small doses over long periods of time. It also is an oxidant, which means it raises the *Oxidation Reduction Potential* (ORP) of anything it comes in contact with, including your body if you drink it. Since chlorine is an oxidant, it *oxidizes,* meaning it *deteriorates* and *ages* the body.

Chlorine also disrupts digestion because it destroys the *Lactobacillus*, the friendly bacteria in the stomach, which retards the intake of nutrients. Like any foreign chemical substance, it also disrupts enzyme reactions which further impedes digestion and overall health. The ammonia that is also commonly added to municipal water reacts unfavorably with the chlorine to form other unwanted substances.

Municipal water should always be carbon filtered before drinking or bathing in. Most Water Ionizers have combination carbon/particulate filters built into them. Showering in unfiltered municipal water can be quite dangerous since the body absorbs more chlorine gas through the skin pores and lungs during a hot shower than it would if you were to drink an eight ounce glass of the same water. Skin pores absorb substances such as chlorine up to twelve times the normal rate in a hot shower because the pores are fully dilated.

The great potential hazard regarding municipal water comes from bacteria such as those that are found only in surface water. Fertilizer, pesticide and other chemical run-off also pose potential problems for municipal water. Ground water has sometimes been found to have volatile organic chemicals (VOC's), such as benzene and trihalomethanes.

Softened Water

(Salt or Potassium Conditioned)

Never drink water than has been run through a salt water softener. Salt softening exchanges the existing minerals in water and replaces them with twice as much salt because of the two to one ion exchange ratio between sodium and other alkaline minerals. Drinking salt-softened water will throw the body's metabolism out of balance and send your blood pressure soaring.

Some believe it is better to drink water softened with potassium chloride instead of sodium chloride because you can drink it. Although potassium is needed by the body more than sodium, potassium chloride has an abundance of chloride, which is an acidic mineral. Although the body needs chloride, it should not be consumed in abundance. For this reason, I recommend not drinking potassium softened water.

Magnetic Water Conditioning

Magnetic water conditioners essentially achieve what a salt or potassium softened water does without the need to put either of them in the water. People often spend between $1000 - $4000 for a salt water softener and then have the burden and expense of endlessly lugging heavy bags of salt for the rest of their lives. What a deal!

Magnetic water conditioners use two very strong South Pole magnets that repel one another. One pair attaches around the water pipe where it enters the house, the other pair around the pipe just after the hot water heater. These powerful magnets polarize the minerals in the water so they line up with one other and will no longer deposit themselves on the interior of the pipe wall. Thus, there is absolutely no pipe scaling whatsoever.

This polarization of minerals in the water actually descales existing deposits on the interior pipe wall. A slow, but steady removal of scaling will occur on areas such as tubs, sinks, etc. If a pipe has significant deposits where scaling has narrowed the interior size of the pipe, magnetic water conditioners will actually open the inner diameter of the pipe over time by descaling it with the polarization effect of the deposited minerals. Like salt softened water, magnetically conditioned water will provide you with more soap lather in the shower, less spotting on dishes and less need for dish and laundry detergent.

Magnetic water conditioners do not add or remove anything from the water. They will not solve iron problems of any kind, which are often caused by house plumbing or old well casings, not source water. They simply polarize the existing minerals that are in the water and change the water's surface tension. They sell for a few hundred dollars, take five minutes to install and usually often come with a twenty-year guaranty.

Chapter 2

Ionized Water

Alkaline Water, Alkalized Water, Cluster Water, Microcluster Water, Reduced Water, Miracle Water, Micro Water, Electrolyzed Water

"Life is a struggle, not against sin, not against money or power, not against malicious animal magnetism, but against hydrogen ions"
-- H.L. Mencken

Alkaline Ionized Water is by far the most superior drinking water available. Ionized Water is electronically enhanced water created through electrolysis. It is produced by running normal tap water over positive and negative electrodes, which ionizes the minerals in the water. The electrodes are composed of titanium and coated with platinum, which is an excellent and durable conductor. It is important to note that the platinum is not electroplated, but coated onto the titanium, meaning it is dipped in the platinum. The membranes are composed of complex polymers. The magic comes when the membranes separate the hydrogen and hydroxyl ions, thus creating alkaline and acidic water. These two waters are produced simultaneously during the ionizing process, 70% Alkaline Water and 30% Acid Water.

To *ionize* simply means to gain or lose an electron. Essentially, the ionization process robs an electron from one molecule and donates, or transfers it another molecule. The molecule that now carries an extra electron is known as a hydroxyl ion, which in this case is an oxygen molecule with an extra electron (See *Antioxidant Section*). It is the presence of hydroxyl ions that makes the water alkaline, meaning it has a high pH.

The other water produced during the ionization process contains hydrogen atom (H+) that have been robbed of an electron. These are known as hydrogen ions and they are what makes the water acid, meaning it has a low pH. (See *Acid Ionized Water* Section).

Both Alkaline and Acid *Ionized Water* have extraordinary properties and benefits, however, their respective uses could not be more different. The Alkaline Water, we drink. The Acid water, we use on the outside of our bodies as well as for many other purposes.

Ionized Water has a beneficial effect on everything it comes in contact with as long as it is used properly. For instance, we should not consume the acid water because it is an oxidant and we would be drinking *free radicals,* unstable oxygen molecules that damage our cells.

Bacteria do not live in Alkaline *Ionized Water* much more than 30-40 seconds because it is an oxygen rich environment and the water has a negative charge, which is hostile to bacteria. Bacteria are killed instantly in Acid *Ionized Water.*

Fresh Alkaline *Ionized Water* that we drink provides the body with huge amounts of negative hydroxyl ions, which negates these hydrogen ions, or *free radicals.* Acidity is measured by the presence of hydrogen ions. The more hydrogen ions that are present, the more acid the water becomes since pH (*potential for hydrogen*) is a measurement of the presence or absence of hydrogen ions.

Hydrogen ions cause oxidation and decay. Free radical molecules are unstable because they are missing an electron. They damage the DNA of a cell when they steal an electron from it. If the cell does not die, it will reproduce using a corrupted set of DNA instructions. Thus both cells will be slightly mutated as if a few critical pages of an instruction manual had been altered or entirely removed. These mutated cells with the now incomplete and/or damaged DNA instructions are the cause of many diseases for obvious reasons. If cells are not replicated with the correct human genetic code, the body now has cells in it that are foreign to its natural state, which is a detriment to the whole body. *Negating hydrogen ions with hydroxyl ions in the* body will retard the onset of disease, as well as the aging process itself. "Because active oxygen can damage normal tissue, it is essential to scavenge this active oxygen from the body before it can cause disintegration of healthy tissue. If we can find an effective method to block the oxidation of healthy tissue by active oxygen, then we can attempt to prevent disease."[10] This is accomplished by drinking *Ionized Water.*

Ionized Water boils and cools about 20-25% faster than conventional water, primarily because of its smaller molecule cluster size and because of the presence of ions in the water, which actually lightens its molecular weight considerable. *Ionized Water* possesses a kind of inexplicable buoyancy. If nothing else, it demonstrates the unusual nature of water that has been ionized.

Ionized Water is one of the most significant preventative health advances of our generation. This is an intentionally profound statement because *Ionized Water* is one of the most beneficial substances available to the human body. As far as importance and impact in my lifetime, it ranks with the first moon-walk and the advent of the personal computer.

Ionized Water is a **Powerful Antioxidant** that provides the body with an abundance of oxygen, which gives us energy. It possesses a negative charge, which is also an antioxidant. It **balances the body's pH**, which helps prevent disease because it is **alkaline**. It is a **Powerful Detoxifier** and **Superior Hydrator,** up to six times more hydrating than conventional water.

Powerful Antioxidant

Negatively Charged Water

The centerpiece of Ionized Water is its antioxidant properties. It is miraculous that normal tap water can be instantly transformed into a strong antioxidant. Ionized Water has two antioxidant qualities, its negative charge and the presence of hydroxyl ions.

All liquids have an Oxidation Reduction Potential (ORP), which is the millivoltage (mV) or vibrational frequency it possesses.

It is said that water has a memory, meaning that it always retains the same ORP unless an external force such as distillation, ionization or other reactive forces change it.

Normal tap water has an ORP of +300 to +400 mV. Its potential for reducing oxidation is nonexistent because its ORP is above zero. Any number over zero indicates that oxidation is occurring. The higher the ORP, the more oxidation is occurring. At +600 mV (+/-) bacteria begin to die. +1100 mV is considered anti-microbial, meaning that bacteria absolutely cannot survive in such a highly charged ORP environment because it literally electrocutes them.

Only a negative ORP can reduce or negate oxidation. Strong Alkaline *Ionized Water* has an ORP of -150 mV to -350 mV, depending on the source water and how many minerals it contains. This low negative number means that the water has a very high potential for reducing oxidation. A -350 mV is better to drink than -150 mV because it negates oxidation of the body more effectively.

Fresh squeezed orange juice has about a -250 mV. All fresh squeezed juices and vegetables have a negative ORP to some degree. Therefore, they are considered antioxidants because they reduce the potential for oxidation. However, if these juices have been heat-treated, pasteurized or otherwise processed, the negative ORP antioxidant properties have been removed from the food. In fact, all its rejuvenation properties have been removed and now the food has become mere sustenance. Enzymes must be present in a food for it to truly be considered rejuvenating. This same principle is true for *Ionized Water*: if it is heated, it will quickly lose its negative charge, although its other properties such as alkalinity and reduce water-cluster size remain intact to some degree. Regardless, *Ionized Water* enhances all foods when cooking with it.

As things oxidize, the ORP rises. Rust is metal that has oxidized. In the human body, oxidation is caused in part by free radical oxidation damage. This means unstable oxygen molecules are robbing us of electrons and this causes oxidation, which leads to aging and disease. As we age, our body's ORP continually rises because we are oxidizing faster. Alkaline *Ionized Water* has a negative ORP; therefore it offsets the positive ORP of our oxidizing, or aging body. Thus, we counteract the aging process by putting a negatively charged substance, which dampens the positive ORP of our oxidizing body. Realistically, we need to drink at least 1 to 2 gallons of strong Alkaline *Ionized Water* per day in order to expect significant slowing and reversal of the aging process.

Increased Oxygen

A fresh glass of strong Alkaline *Ionized Water* right out of the tap will contain a cloud of tiny bubbles in the water. These are hydroxyl ions, *Ionized Water's* other antioxidant component. This is the best way to drink *Ionized Water*, as fresh as possible.

To *Ionize* means to gain or lose an electron. In the case of *Ionized Water*, an electron is grabbed from one hydrogen atom and donated to a oxygen molecule, which then becomes a hydroxyl ion: an oxygen molecule with an extra electron. As a result, has become an antioxidant capable of scavenging for free radicals in the body and negating them before they cause damage.

"Oxygen is essential to survival. It is relatively stable in the air, but when too much is absorbed into the body it can become active and unstable and has a tendency to attach itself to any biological molecule, including molecules of healthy cells. The chemical activity of these free radicals is due to one or more pairs of unpaired electrons . . . Such free radicals with unpaired electrons are unstable and have a high oxidation potential, which means they are capable of stealing electrons from other cells." [11]

Some antioxidants possess an extra electron, others do not. *Ionized Water* is an extremely effective antioxidant because it is a liquid with small water molecule clusters and thus is more easily absorbed into the body where it can be of immediate use.

Antioxidants have anti-aging and anti-disease properties because they help return the body's cells to a healthier, youthful, natural state. *Ionized Water* is a liquid antioxidant; therefore, it is extremely effective and more easily absorbed into the body than any other antioxidant. As we make *Ionized Water* a part of our daily routine and drink sufficient quantities of it, we begin to bathe the body's cells in alkalinity and antioxidants, while at the same time better hydrating them than they have ever been. Nothing could be more fundamentally better for our health.

"When taken internally, the reduced ionized water with its redox potential (ORP) of -250 to -350 mV readily donates its electrons to oddball oxygen radicals and blocks the interaction of the active oxygen with normal molecules." [12]

Essentially, all disease appears and develops in the body from either the environment or diet, unless it is congenital in nature, meaning genetically inherited or a condition that exists at birth. Environmental diseases may come from artificial sources such as chemical toxins, naturally occurring toxic substances, or even insect-borne diseases.

Free radicals are another example of the environment encouraging disease in our body by causing cell mutations and other types of cellular damage. Free radical cell damage is a big part of the aging equation.

"Problems arise, however, when too many of these active oxygen molecules, or free radicals, are produced in the body. They are extremely reactive and can also attach themselves to normal, healthy cells and damage them genetically. These active oxygen radicals steal electrons from normal, healthy biological molecules. This electron theft by active oxygen oxidizes tissue and can cause disease." [13]

Drinking Ionized Water gives you energy. On the surface, it seems like an outrageous claim that drinking water could possibly give a person energy. However, strong, fresh *Ionized Water* possesses an abundance of hydroxyl ions, which destroy free radicals by donating an electron to them and leaving behind two stabilized oxygen molecules, thus providing the body with more oxygen. Check your blood oxygen level before you first start drinking *Ionized Water* and then again a few weeks after you have been drinking it regularly and see the difference for yourself.

Energy derived from oxygen is the best form of energy a person can have because it has not been derived from an artificial source such as caffeine, sugar or other chemical stimulants. These substances produce an artificial energy rush that eventually lets us down once they are used up. For instance, when we consume too much sugar, the pancreas produces insulin to counteract the sudden influx of excess sugar, and we experience a sugar/insulin crash. Years of doing this can eventually lead to diabetes, one of several diseases that have become epidemic among children because of their high sugar, processed food diet.

However, with oxygen, it's an entirely different story. The body never gets a rush from oxygen and never crashes from it because it is naturally derived energy. It picks us up slowly and let us down slowly as it is used up. People who drink *Ionized Water* on a regular basis don't notice how much energy it gives them until the fourth or fifth day after they stop drinking it and the oxygen-induced energy has finally dissipated.

Oxygen is a nutrient the body desperately needs. It makes us alert and invigorated. It carries vital nutrients around the body. The body cannot store oxygen because oxygen has a blood saturation level and the body quickly discards any surplus. This is important because we must constantly provide the body with more oxygen and there is no better natural source than *Ionized Water*. Millions of years ago there was as much as 30% more oxygen in the atmosphere, therefore we evolved over billions of years in a richer oxygen environment than there is on Earth today.

For someone with cancer, the high oxygen level provided by *Ionized Water* is particularly helpful since oxygen destroys cancer cells. Cancer patients are often tired because their blood oxygen levels are low after being depleted by the process of mutual destruction between cancer cells and oxygen molecules. By drinking strong *Ionized Water* on a regular basis the amount of oxygen in the blood will increase. This is helpful in fighting many diseases since oxygen is a poison to both cancer and bacteria; therefore the more we can get into our blood stream, the better.

"There is no substitute for a healthy balanced diet, especially rich in antioxidant materials such as vitamin C, vitamin E, beta-carotene, and other foods that are good for us. However, these substances are not the best source of free electrons that can block the oxidation of healthy tissue by active oxygen. Water treated by electrolysis to increase its reduction potential is the best solution to the problem of providing a safe source of free electrons to block the oxidation of normal tissue by free oxygen radicals. We believe that reduced water, water with an excess of free electrons to donate to active oxygen, is the best solution . . ." [14]

Balances Body pH

Because of the predominance of hydroxyl ions in *Ionized Water*, the water becomes alkaline, meaning it has a high pH. The pH level can be adjusted with a Water Ionizer between 7 and 10. At a 10 pH, *Ionized Water* begins to taste briny, so there is a limit to how strong *Ionized Water* should be consumed even though it is not harmful to drink over a 10 pH. A 9.5 to 9.9 pH is sufficiently strong enough to satisfy the body's needs for oxygen, alkalinity, a negative ORP, hydroxyl ions and proper hydration.

The ease at which a 10 pH or higher is achieved will depend on how slow the water runs through the Water Ionizer, what the water temperature is and how high the mineral content is. *The more minerals in the source water, the stronger Ionized Water will be.* Some Water Ionizers have built-in mineral ports where calcium and other water soluble minerals can be leached into, or added, to the water as it passes through the filter before it is ionized. Purified water, either distilled or by reverse osmosis, has no mineral content and therefore *no ionization would occur* if this water was used with a Water Ionizer.

"Alkaline water, having a pH of between 9 and 11, will neutralize harmful stored acid wastes, and if you consume it every day, will gently remove them from your body. Yet, since the water is ionized, it will not leach out valuable minerals like calcium, magnesium, potassium, or sodium." [15]

There are both alkaline minerals and acid minerals. Ionization will become stronger on the alkaline side if there are mostly alkaline minerals present in the water and stronger on the acid side if there are mostly acid minerals present.

Alkaline Minerals: Calcium, magnesium, sodium, potassium and manganese are known as alkaline-forming minerals because they have a positive charge. These minerals will strengthen the alkaline side of the *Ionized Water* by forming more hydroxyl ions.

". . . all ingested substances and all situations (physical, emotional, or mental) that affect the body, leave either an alkaline or acid ash residue in the urine."[16] For instance, each time the heart beats it uses magnesium. The residual magnesium ash comes out in the urine and is easily discarded if the body is balanced and healthy.

Acid Minerals: Sulfur, iodine, chlorine, phosphorous, bromine, copper, silicon and fluoride are known as acid-forming minerals because they have a negative charge. The body uses many acid minerals, which leaves acid ash behind when they are used up. The presence of these minerals will strengthen the acid side of the *Ionized Water* by forming more hydrogen ions. The body removes ash efficiently when it is healthy and balanced.

The fact that the *Ionized Water* we drink is alkaline is very important because *disease thrives in an acidic environment and will not flourish and thrive in an Alkaline environment.* Thus, if someone creates an acidic environment in the body by years of eating acid foods and/or putting other acid substances in the bodies such as drugs, alcohol, cigarettes, soft drinks, processed sugar, etc., then they become vulnerable to any disease that invades the body, regardless of the source. The more acidic a person is, the more susceptible they are to disease. As disease flourishes in the body, it begins to create a more acidic environment in order to spread further until it consumes the body.

"Living things are extremely sensitive to pH and function best (with certain exceptions, such as certain portions of the digestive tract) when solutions are nearly neutral. Most interior living matter (excluding the cell nucleus) has a pH of about 6.8." [17]

When some cancer patients are near death, their bodies begin to produce ammonia as a natural chemical reaction meant to counteract the extremely acidic environment that has been created in their body by the cancer. This is the bad odor that some cancer victims have as they near death.

"Therefore, in my opinion, acid wastes literally attack the joints, tissues, muscles, organs and glands causing minor to major dysfunction." [Sic] [18] Currently, the medical establishment as a whole has not embraced the idea that body pH and disease work hand in hand. The fact is that if you have a cold or flu you will feel much better after raising the pH of your body by drinking *Ionized Water* and eating as many fresh fruits, vegetables and herbs as you can. Drinking herbal tea with fresh lemon will often make you feel better when you're sick because lemon is a strong alkaloid, meaning that it creates a great deal of alkalinity in the body when consumed. By raising its pH, the body is given its best chance to fight the virus, bacteria or other disease that has invaded it with the defenses it has in its arsenal. We call this our immune system, which functions optimally when the body is balanced.

Body alkalinity is most accurately measured through the saliva or urine. One of the keys to Great Health is keeping the body pH properly balanced and alkaline. Drinking plenty of *Ionized Water* will help achieve that.

Powerful Detoxifier and Superior Hydrator

Ionized Water is sometimes called *Reduced Water* or *Cluster Water* because of its small molecular grouping. Water molecules typically group together in clusters of 10-13. *Ionized Water* molecule clusters are split in half and clustered into 5-6 water molecules, thus they are *reduced* in size. The *Ionized Water* molecule cluster also has been changed from an irregular shape to a *regular, hexagonal shape* that passes through and saturates body tissue much more efficiently than conventional water. It is this smaller, regular shaped cluster that hydrates everything it comes in contact with.

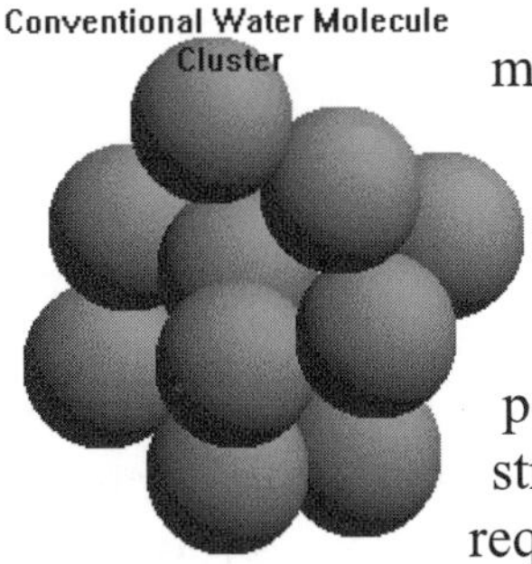

Conventional Water Molecule Cluster

All Water Ionizers currently manufactured have more than one level of ionization strength. Some of the older models have only one level, which is quite limiting when it comes to adjusting the pH level of *Ionized Water.* And this is critical to many people when they first start drinking it. The strong detoxification aspects of *Ionized Water* requires that some people begin by drinking it rather weak, then slowly building the strength of the *Ionized Water* over time until they acclimate to it. Headaches, rashes and diarrhea are common detoxification symptoms when first using *Ionized Water.* Quality Ionized Waters have four or five levels of strength, which allows people to slowly ease into *Ionized Water* when they first start drinking it in order to mollify these detoxification effects that can be quite dramatic for those who are toxic.

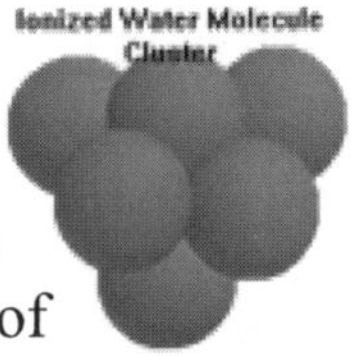

Ionized Water Molecule Cluster

One reason the side affects of detoxification are so strong is because as the *Ionized Water* so efficiently hydrates body tissue with its micro-cluster structure. This penetrating water leaves less room for anything else in the tissue. Thus the toxins are effectively pushed out of the tissue and into the bloodstream to then be eliminated by the body.

We cannot drink too much *Ionized Water* once the body has acclimated to it. But the more toxins a person has in their body, the weaker the *Ionized Water* should be at the start so the detoxification effects are kept to a minimum. In general, the level of *Ionized Water* a person should start drinking depends on what kind of shape they keep themselves in, meaning how toxic they are. If a person maintains a good diet, drinks a lot of water, doesn't smoke, drink heavily, take drugs or medication, they can usually start by drinking *Ionized Water* on one of the higher levels of strength.

Regarding children, the vast majority of them have no trouble drinking *Ionized Water* on the strongest level at the start because they are too young to have accumulated many toxins in their bodies. Since they are young, their bodies produce many times more enzymes than adults do and this also allows their bodies to quickly adjust to *Ionized Water.*

However, it is just the opposite with the elderly who have a lifetime of toxins and heavy metals accumulated in their bodies and are often on medications that also need to be detoxified, or removed.

Drinking *Ionized Water* while you are taking medications will not interfere with the function of those medications. However, the medications themselves should **not** be taken with *Ionized Water* because it will cause the medication to enter the body very quickly and some medications are designed to be time released. Thus, caution should be exercised in this regard. Always consult your doctor when taking medication with any liquid other than conventional water.

When consumed, *Ionized Water* moves through the body rather quickly, up to 30% faster than conventional water. Acid *Ionized Water,* however, moves through the body rather slowly if consumed, which is an indication that its effects on the body are opposite of Alkaline *Ionized Water.*

Ionized Water is up to six times more hydrating than conventional water. It is easy to demonstrate the effects of *Ionized Water* regarding its smaller molecule cluster and superior hydration. Soaking things such as dried kidney or pinto beans in *Ionized Water* will cause them to hydrate considerably faster and swell fatter. Mixing *Ionized Water* with any kind of powder or flour will result in much better absorption than using conventional water. For instance, making gravy or cream soup with *Ionized Water* will result in a smoother texture and no lumpiness, which is further evidence that the absorption factor of *Ionized Water* regarding any material is greater compared to conventional water.

Cooking with *Ionized Water* will enhance the taste of the food because of this hydrating, swelling effect. The minerals and other nutrients in the food will also be assimilated into the body more efficiently because they have been ionized.

Allergies and Ionized Water

Ionized Water can be of significant help to allergy sufferers. Drinking *Ionized Water* will help keep the body alkaline, well hydrated and cleansed with detoxifying water that flushes accumulated pollen, mold and chemical substances from the body.

People who suffer from sneezing, itchy eyes, scratchy throat, etc. during allergy season should use Alkaline *Ionized Water* to flush the eyes, nose, mouth, throat, ears and face in order to stop itching, scratchiness and irritation. Alkaline *Ionized Water* is effective in such instances because these types of seasonal allergies are caused by pollen, which is part of a plant, and Alkaline *Ionized Water* retards plant growth.

Since Acid *Ionized Water* enhances plant growth, the result of applying Acid *Ionized Water* to the eyes and other areas that are itchy or irritated due to pollen is to actually invigorate or waken the pollen, thus making the condition worse. It is the hydrogen ions in Acid *Ionized Water* that causes this rejuvenation and conditioning of the pollen. Flushing the eyes and other affected areas instead with Alkaline *Ionized Water* has the opposite effect of allaying the allergic condition by suppressing the activity of the pollen.

The Benefits of Alkaline Water

High pH - (Hydroxyl Ions)
(Drinking Water)

Gives you energy!

- **Provides the body with lots of oxygen**
- **Removes accumulated acid waste and toxins from the body**
- **Promotes overall health and healing by bringing the body into pH balance**
- **Retards the aging process with its negative charge**
- **Hydrates the body up to six times more effectively than conventional water**
- **Foods cooked with *Ionized Water* taste better and are more healthy**
- **Minerals that are ionized are more easily assimilated by the body**
- **Powders such as flour are mixed more thoroughly and smoothly**

- **Promotes regularity and digestive health by internally cleansing the body**
- **Helps relieve seasonal allergies**

Acid Ionized Water

The Other Half of Unbelievable

Having Acid Ionized Water on tap is worth the price of a Water Ionizer in and of itself because of its extraordinary uses and benefits. Acid *Ionized Water* is an oxidant. When Acid *Ionized Water* is freshly produced, small bubbles are present in the water, but not as many as on the alkaline side, which tends to be far more cloudy with hydroxyl ions. However, the bubbles on the acid side are hydrogen ions, which are free radicals: unstable molecules that are missing an electron. **For that reason, we should NEVER drink Acid *Ionized Water.***

Acid *Ionized Water* kills bacteria on contact. How much it kills depends on the strength of the acid water, i.e., how high the ORP (mV) and how low the pH is. For instance, an ORP 1100 mV and a 2.5 pH is considered anti-microbial, meaning that it kills all bacteria on contact. By comparison, chlorine, which is also an oxidant, has a one second bacterial kill rate at 700 mV. Mild Acid *Ionized Water* produced from tap water using a home Water Ionizer has a range of 700-950 mV, depending on the source water, which is quite effective at killing bacteria.

In Japan, Acid *Ionized Water* is used effectively on golf courses as a combination fertilizer and pesticide. Acid *Ionized Water* has a very nice conditioning effect on the skin and hair because they both are also somewhat acid, which is the body's first line of defense against bacteria. The skin has about a 4.7 pH, the hair about 5.6 pH.

Applying Ionized Acid Water regularly to the skin works as an astringent to tighten it and remove wrinkles; however, there is NO chemical residue as there is with other skin moisteners and conditioners. In fact, there is no residue at all. Acid *Ionized Water* soothes and helps keep the skin clear of acne and other blemishes. Since acne is caused by bacteria, Acid *Ionized Water* helps destroy the cause of the acne; and because of its smaller molecule cluster size, it is able to penetrate into the skin better to kill the bacteria. Combined with drinking *Ionized Water*, conditions such as these will improve greatly.

The more Acid *Ionized Water* is applied on the skin and hair, the better they respond, and there is no limit to the number of applications a person can have in a day. Skin and hair, even animal fur, respond very positively to the conditioning effects of Acid *Ionized Water*.

Acid *Ionized Water* improves hair and skin conditions of all kinds such as eczema, psoriasis, cuts, scrapes, skin ulcers, even serious wounds, as well as athlete's feet and other fungus. It takes the itch out of mosquito bites and the sting out of other insect bites. It provides relief from poison oak and poison ivy exposure. It will even take down the swelling of a fat lip.

Scalp problems such as dandruff are improved with Acid *Ionized Water*. Along with eating a proper diet comprised of *Spirulina*, *Chlorella,* fresh fruits and vegetables, as well as drinking Alkaline *Ionized Water*, many of these health problems can be eliminated entirely because they are an indication that we are lacking key nutrients in our diet.

Skin tissue heals better with the use of Acid *Ionized Water*. It has been used successfully in treating diabetic skin ulcers, which are wounds that open up in the skin of a diabetic and are notoriously difficult to heal because they will not cauterize nor properly drain. Diabetics sometimes must have feet and even legs amputated because the ulcers become infected and gangrene beyond treatment. However, soaking ulcers in Acid *Ionized Water* has a tremendous healing effect on them. It kills the bacteria around the wound and allows it to cauterize so it can then heal. Doctors insist that diabetic ulcers must be kept absolutely dry at all times, yet Acid *Ionized Water* is an effective treatment that breaks that rule! Medical professionals are at a loss to explain the success of using water to treat diabetic ulcers.

Drinking Alkaline *Ionized Water* is a great benefit to diabetics because it helps bring the body into pH balance and provides it with lots of oxygen. This helps carry nutrients around the body and further brings the body into balance, which is key to fighting any disease.

Acid *Ionized Water* makes plants grow extremely well. Its low pH properties are quite favorable to plants that usually thrive best if the soil is slightly acidic. The adjustability of the pH on a Water Ionizer is helpful in this regard. The smaller molecule clusters of Acid *Ionized*

Water transpire into the plant much more effectively than conventional water, which helps increase the turgor of the plant. Acid *Ionized Water* contains hydrogen ions as do most fertilizers. Thus, feeding Acid *Ionized Water* to a plant has a similar effect to that of fertilizing it.

The difference between feeding a plant Acid *Ionized Water* and conventional water is profound. When plants are fed Acid *Ionized Water*, it soon becomes apparent when a plant first started receiving the superior water by the healthier growth from that exact point on the plant on up. Overall, plants fed Acid *Ionized Water* look much healthier, its flowers brighter, its leaves shinier and darker green.

Another demonstration of Acid *Ionized Water's* power is to place two oranges side by side and spray one with Acid *Ionized Water* three or four times a day and not the other. The orange that is not sprayed with Acid *Ionized Water* will decay much quicker than the one sprayed with the Acid *Ionized Water*, which will last several days longer. This demonstrates the claim that Acid *Ionized Water* kills bacteria as it does on the sprayed orange, thus allowing it to decay more slowly than the one that was not sprayed.

If acid minerals such as phosphorous or chloride are not in great abundance in the source water that is being ionized, the pH of the Acid *Ionized Water* will not drop significantly. However, even without the presence of a low pH (6.5 +/-), Acid *Ionized Water* is quite effective.

Benefits of Acid *Ionized Water*

Low pH - (Hydrogen Ions)

EXTERNAL USE ONLY - Do not Drink

Kills bacteria on contact

Helps heal cuts, blisters, scrapes, rashes, burns, serious wounds

Helps heal diabetic skin ulcers

Provides relief from mosquito bites and bee stings

Provides relief from poison ivy and poison oak

Cleans and conditions hair

Great for car, truck or boat batteries

Excellent astringent skin conditioner

Relieves chapped hands & dry, itchy skin

Effectively removes plaque from teeth. Use it instead of toothpaste

Wash vegetables, fruits, meats and fish with it to kill bacteria

Gargle with it to relieve sore throats and mouth sores

Acts as an astringent to tighten skin and remove wrinkles

Excellent treatment for acne, eczema and other skin and scalp diseases

Excellent treatment for fungus such as athletes foot

Excellent cleaning agent

Promotes healthy plant growth
Significantly extends the life of cut flowers

Super Acid Ionized Water

Super Acid Water Ionizers produce very strong Ionized Acid Water with an ORP of 1100 mV and a 2.5 pH. This is achieved by using stronger electrodes and by adding pure salt (sodium chloride) to the water, which drives up the pH on the alkaline side and drives down the pH on the acid side. Sodium is an alkaline mineral, chloride is an acid mineral. By using the sodium to raise the pH of *Ionized Water* on the alkaline side and chloride on the acid side, the result is very strong forms of both Acid *Ionized Water* and Alkaline *Ionized Water.* Super Alkaline *Ionized Water*, with a pH of 14(+/-) is an excellent degreaser.

Super Acid *Ionized Water,* or HOP (High Oxidation Potential) Water, is used primarily for medicinal purposes, such as for advanced diabetic ulcers, serious wounds or burns.

At a 2.5 pH, it is antimicrobial, meaning that it kills all bacteria on contact. It is far too strong for immediate contact with most plants and needs to be slightly diluted. Super Acid *Ionized Water* could be used as a hand disinfectant in hospitals where 80% of all people who are infected while in the hospital contract their disease by way of doctors and nurses not washing their hands between patient visits.

It could also be used with livestock, especially on newborns, which would promote a cleaner environment, helping to lower veterinary costs and mortality rates. Unfortunately, Super Acid Water Ionizers tend to be quite costly. They are typically meant for commercial operations and have limited practical uses in the average household.

Ionized Water is for Everyone

Ionized Water benefits everyone who drinks it. To get the full benefits of *Ionized Water*, one should drink it fresh from the tap and as strong as possible. There are few retail locations in North America that sell *Ionized Water* by the gallon. Having *Ionized Water* on tap is well worth the investment in your health. Water Ionizers are currently manufactured only in Korea and Japan. There are several Water Ionizer models available on the market and most of them offer comparable performance, although retail prices can vary widely. Units that have a fuse instead of a circuit breaker tend to come with bigger transformers, thus they have less of a tendency to overheat or surge and trip the fuse. One thing to look for is whether the unit has more than one level. Water Ionizers are analogous to toasters in that prices may range from $20 - $120 for a toaster; however, regardless of how much you pay, you still simply end up with toast.

Korean Water Ionizers are generally less expensive than Japanese models and their quality in recent years now rivals Japanese manufacturing. Buying a Water Ionizer with an ultra violet (UV) light to disinfect the water on its way into the unit is a waste of money because UV light is unnecessary in most cases, expensive and ineffective after only a few months of use because the tube that carries the water clouds up.

There are a few companies bottling *Ionized Water,* which is usually sold in health food stores. However, bottling *Ionized Water* is erroneous because the Antioxidant, the centerpiece of *Ionized Water*, is long gone by the time it reaches the shelf, as is most of the alkalinity. Bottled *Ionized Water* tastes a little smoother than conventional water because some of the reduced molecule clusters will linger for months after it is bottled. However, the overall strength of bottled *Ionized Water* is only a fraction of the power of fresh *Ionized Water* out of the tap.

Ionized Water and Fluoride Removal

It has been suggested that Water Ionizers remove 100% of all the fluoride in the source water by sending it all down the drain by way of the acid water tube because fluoride is an acid mineral. 100% fluoride removal through ionization is a physical impossibility since 100% of the water would need to be ionized to remove 100% of any mineral either to the alkaline or acid water tubes. Tests consistently demonstrate that the removal rate of fluoride through the Acid *Ionized Water* side is approximately 45-50%, which means that about half of the fluoride in the water will be removed to the acid side at the highest (strongest) ionization level.

How Long Ionized Water Lasts

Ionized Water is not very stable. The best way to store it is in a cool dark place. Keep it out of the sunlight because the ultra violet rays will react with the water and quickly weaken it. If stored in a container, it will lose its strength more quickly once opened and exposed to the air.

Anything reacting with it will cause it to lose its ionized condition and it will revert back to conventional water.

Hydroxyl Ions: 10 - 20 minutes of effectiveness
(A small number will remain up to 24 hours)

Negative ORP (mV charge): 18-24 hours

Alkalinity (high pH): 3 - 8 days

Smaller molecule clusters: 2 - 3 months

Acid *Ionized Water*: 30-180 days in a cool, dark place, undisturbed.

How Much to Drink

I drink approximately two gallons of *Ionized Water* everyday and have never felt better. The benefits of drinking *Ionized Water* are profound regarding their effect on the human body. Since it provides the body with an abundance of oxygen, it gives me lots of energy. My body pH is balanced around 7.0 where it should be. My muscles are more relaxed because much of the lactic acid waste has been washed from the muscle tissue. I am over 40 and do not ache in any of my joints. I am undoubtedly more limber, oxygenated, detoxified, and better hydrated than anytime in my life.

If I feel a cold or flu coming on, a glass or two of *Ionized Water* helps put it in check because my body is fully accustomed to receiving the oxygen released from drinking *Ionized Water*.

I was in my late thirties when I started drinking *Ionized Water* and thirty-eight years of accumulated acid waste deposited throughout the human body takes months, even years to remove. It will take a lot of water and lot of time to fully accomplish the goal of complete pH balance and detoxification throughout my body.

Installation & Use

Water Ionizers come with a faucet diverter and about three feet of tubing. To install the unit, remove the aerator on the sink faucet and replace it with the diverter. Cut the single length of tubing in half and attach one piece from the diverter into the inlet of the Water Ionizer. The other piece of tubing attaches where the Acid *Ionized Water* exits the unit and drapes into the sink. The Alkaline *Ionized Water* exits the unit from a stainless steel tube on top of the unit.

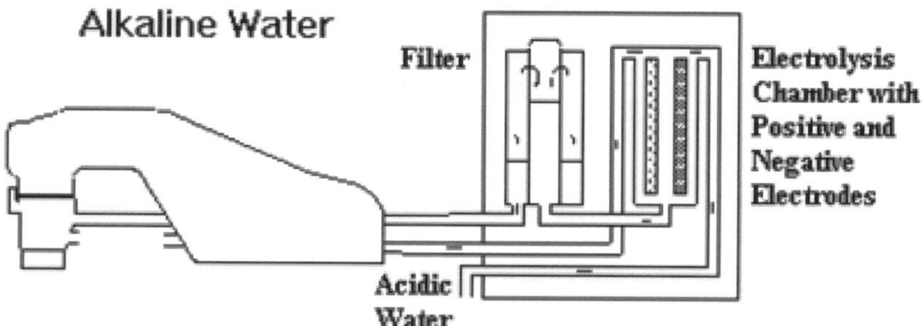

Acid *Ionized Water* can be collected for use at a later time, although, like Alkaline *Ionized Water*, the fresher it is, the stronger it is.

After several months, the electrodes on a *Water Ionizer* will begin to coat with minerals such as calcium, which will reduce the strength of the *Ionized Water* since the source water is no longer coming in direct contact with the electrodes. Running the unit in cleaning mode will help retard the coating, but it will not entirely stop it from happening. Recirculating vinegar through the unit with a small fish or landscaping pump will clean the electrodes.

Where to Install Your Water Ionizer

Water Ionizers can be installed at any sink in the house, most commonly in the kitchen or bathroom. Jupiter Water Ionizers can sit on the counter or can be hung from wall next to your sink. Two holes in the back of the units are provided for hanging the unit. Water Ionizers will not work properly if one attempts to operate it from underneath your sink.

Water Ionizer Installation

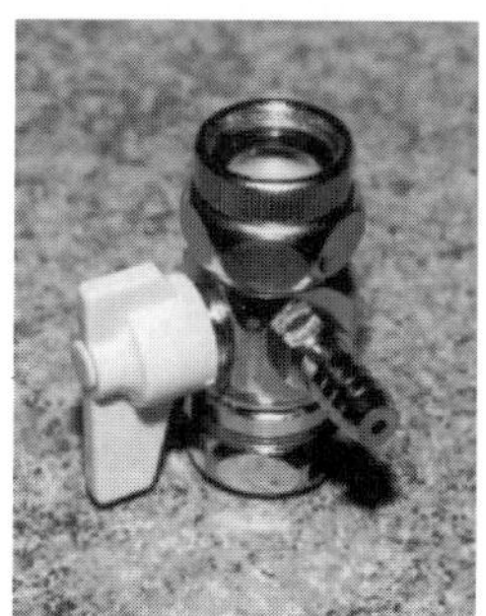

Step 1: Screw in Stainless Steel tube to the top of the unit.
Step 2: Remove aerator from the faucet and attach Faucet Diverter to Faucet.
Step 3: Cut plastic hose in half.
Step 4: Attach one hose to the Faucet Diverter and the other end into the bottom of the Water Ionizer marked INLET.
Step 5: Attach the other hose to the bottom of the Water Ionizer labeled OUTLET and drapes the tube into the sink.
Step 6: Plug the unit into an electrical outlet.*
Step 7: Turn on the faucet and begin running water through the unit.

Typical installation takes approximately 10 minutes and usually does not require a plumber to install.

PART TWO

Chapter 3

Nutrition & Body pH

Health is my expected heaven. -- John Keats

The human body is an intricate mechanism far beyond our current capabilities of fully understanding it. For instance, what microbiologists know today about the human cell compared to what they thought they knew only 20 years ago is staggering. Many notions that were accepted as fact concerning the human cell have been demonstrated to be flat wrong. For instance, how cells communicate with one another, what information is communicated, how it functions, adapts, everything has been relearned and rethought. Everyday we are discovering more about human physiology, and have only scratched the surface.

What is known about certain forms of dementia, especially in the elderly, is minimal, which illustrates how little is known about the human brain and how it actually functions. Although some success has been achieved, treatment for psychiatric disorders such as Lewy Body Dementia, Alzheimer Disease and numerous others are akin to medieval. Diseases such as these are encouraged by toxins accumulating throughout the body and in the brain and from a lifetime of not drinking enough water. It is imperative these toxins are constantly removed throughout our lives.

If we provide the body, and ultimately its cells, with exactly the nutrients it needs, the cells will rebuild themselves, function perfectly and reproduce (divide) with little or no diminution. Essentially, *we are only as healthy as our body's cells.* And they are only healthy when they are properly supplied with the nutrients, *building materials*, they require to function. Our overall health is reflective of our health at a cellular level. The question then becomes *what nutrients should we provide the body's cells with in order for them to function efficiently and to their full capacity?*

Death or Life: Keeping the Body Alkaline & Balanced

"That which is built on alkalinity sustains: That which is built on acidity falls away -- be it civilizations, human bodies, or the paper that preserves their knowledge."

-- Dr. T. Baroody

The world's written history was recorded on alkaline paper until 1850 when it began to be recorded on acid paper. Those original written records starting in 1850 are disintegrating at an alarming rate. The best that can be done is to scan them electronically and save what is left of the books by re-alkalizing the remaining paper. However, books printed on alkaline paper before 1850 still survive, often in perfect condition. Acid destroys life. A balanced, slightly alkaline pH, preserves it.

When discussing body pH, I am referring to the pH measurement of either urine or saliva. It is the only convenient way of gauging overall body pH, and even these measurements can be deceptive if not taken properly.

The liquid that exists between the body's cells is a complicated medium of chemicals known as transcellular fluids. It is a delicate pH balance between alkaline and acid, which must be maintained within a very narrow pH range. Because it is a liquid, any change in its pH can have a profound effect on the body's chemistry, overall health and its ability to effectively fight disease.

If this fluid becomes too acidic, the body's pH management will be thrown out of balance, its severity in direct correlation to the acid level. Body pH regulates circulation, hormonal production and balance, digestion and elimination, the immune system, respiratory system and inter/intracellular communications.

"If the condition of our extracellular fluids, especially the blood, becomes acidic, our physical condition will first manifest tiredness, proneness to catching colds, etc. When these fluids become more acidic, our condition then manifests pains and suffering such as headaches, chest pains, stomach aches, etc." [19]

Three systems control pH in the body: the Urinary System, Respiratory System, and Chemical and Physiological Buffering

System. If the body becomes too acid (a low pH) meaning that it has too many hydrogen ions (H+), the excess acid is immediately removed through the urine. If this acidity becomes a common occurrence in the body, the pH balance control systems can become overburdened, beyond their ability to properly balance the body's pH.

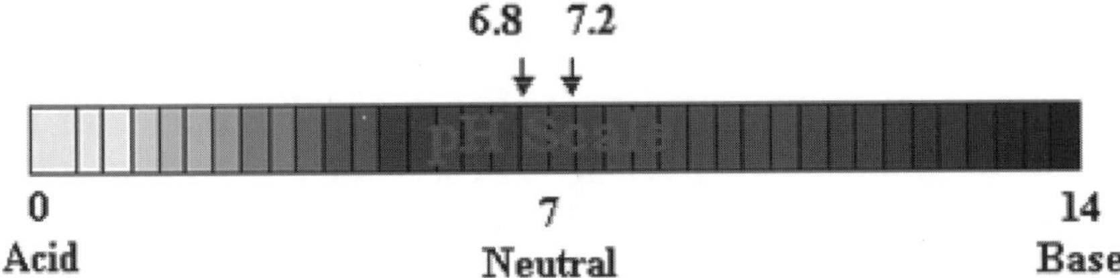

It is vital that our blood plasma remain slightly alkaline, between 7.25 - 7.45 pH. If it falls below 7.25 pH, we develop acidosis, the condition of being too acid, which is common, not often diagnosed, understood nor seen as significant. If it rises above 7.45 pH, we develop *alkalosis*, the condition of being too alkaline, which is quite rare. Either condition is dangerous to the point of being fatal if the pH falls too far out of that narrow range.

As acid waste enters the blood, it is quickly relocated to other parts of the body, collecting primarily in the joints, connective tissue and around the organs. The extracellular fluids, the liquid between cells, become acid. This directly compromises cellular integrity and will eventually acidify the cells themselves. **The body then develops an overall acidic profile, which lays the groundwork for disease to flourish when it attacks.**

The Acid Profile Theory (APT) postulates that many diseases are caused themselves by the body becoming too acid over long periods of time. Broadly speaking, disease arises from one of three places: the environment (allergies, natural or artificial toxic pollutants, viruses, bacteria); genetic origin (inherited); or from poor diet, especially a diet that has replaced fresh fruits and vegetables with processed foods.

Keiichi Morishita says in his book, The Hidden Truth of Cancer, that a high acid body environment causes cell mutation and these malignant cells are unable to properly communicate with other cells, nor are they able to function within the body's predetermined genetic structure. This, Morishita claims, is the beginning of cancer.

Dr. Otto Warburg, in The Metabolism of Tumors, postulates that lack of oxygen to the cell is the root cause of cancer. These theories of acidity and oxygen deprivation being the root cause of diseases have many variations, proponents and detractors. There is most likely truth of be found in all these theories, but add to them enzyme and water deprivation and we move closer to understanding ALL the causes of disease. **Removing sufficient amounts of water and enzymes from the body is a deadly combination that certainly will encourage chronic disease of every kind**.

Nearly all cellular and organ activity in the body is sensitive to pH variation, especially if the pH is well outside the acceptable range. The blood is a perfect example. The kidneys remove more acid from the body than any other organ. However, since the blood transports acid waste to the kidneys, there is a tremendous limit on how much acid the blood can carry at any given time. The blood itself becomes one of the greatest bottlenecks to the entire acid waste removal systems of the body. It is trying to remove excess hydrogen ions (H+), which is essentially what causes something to be acid in the first place. Another problem is that the kidneys will not excrete acid below a 5.4 pH. The body is then forced to store excess amounts of acid waste in its tissue and around the organs because the kidneys cannot handle its removal. Once it is settled in these places it becomes more difficult to remove. Drinking *Ionized Water* can substantially eliminate hydrogen ions and excess acidity in the body if enough is consumed.

Over long periods of time, the toxic nature of the acid will actually begin to poison the cells themselves, especially in areas where it has been deposited in the connective tissue. The dead cells now produce blockages wherever they lay. Whether they dangerously impede cardiovascular passages or the flow of information between cells, nutrients are no longer being supplied as efficiently to the body because of these dead cells.

"The total increment in net acid excretion by the kidneys is often lower than total acid production, resulting in a positive hydrogen-ion imbalance. It has been postulated that bone has an important role in the buffering of long-term acid loads." [20] This would account for osteoporosis and related disease because the bones demonstrate that they have been catalyzed in an acid/alkaline reaction. Cells that have been introduced into a more acid environment will

begin to mutate in order to exist in that more acid environment and cell mutation is never a good thing because mutated cells would be considered outside invaders by the rest of the body.

Lowering the pH of the body dramatically causes many enzymatic reactions to cease thus putting cellular metabolism itself at risk. Enzymes and enzyme reactions are some of the most basic and important functions of the body.

As the acid condition worsens, it destroys cell walls, corroding veins and arteries and eventually entire organs. The skin of an overly acidic person is markedly more wrinkled, worn, unhealthy and more prone to disease compared to someone who is alkaline.

In the purest of terms, pH is a measurement of electrical resistance between negative and positive ions in the human body. If the body possesses an abundance of positive hydrogen ions, we are acidic. If the body possesses an abundance of negative hydroxyl ions, we are alkaline.

It is difficult to measure body pH accurately because so many things can cause the pH of urine or saliva to rise or fall. For instance, consuming something that is extremely alkaline such as asparagus or *Ionized Water* will turn the urine acidic because these substances remove acid waste from the body, even though on balance the body has become more alkaline.

The most accurate urine reading is first thing in the morning. Saliva is also accurate as long as you haven't drank or eaten anything for 45 minutes before taking the pH measurement. We should try to maintain the body pH close to 7.0.

Litmus pH paper is not terribly accurate. Color pH test drops are a little better. For accuracy and reliability a digital pH meter and buffer (calibration) solution is a must. They are good to have around for measuring the pH of *Ionized Water*, other liquids that you consume and the pH of the body itself.

Minerals

Some of the most important elements that the body requires are minerals and it needs them in the correct ratio to one another in order for them to work effectively in the body. Calcium, magnesium, potassium and sodium are called electrolytes because they are conductors. They are the primary minerals the body requires as well as more than 70 other trace minerals, which are used and catalyzed all over the body. Drinking *Ionized Water* is helpful because the body assimilates minerals that have been ionized more efficiently. Some Water Ionizers have a mineral port where calcium and other water-soluble minerals can be added which strengthens the ionization process and results in strong *Ionized Water*. Always use pure minerals with a Water Ionizer, not those that are chelated because they can coat the electrodes.

Just as a spark plug ignites fuel to run an engine, each time the heart beats it uses magnesium to fire, which causes the heart to beat. Insufficient amounts of magnesium in the body will not allow the heart to function properly. If depletion becomes serious enough, it will eventually lead to a heart attack. The first thing most hospitals do when a heart attack victim arrives at a trauma center is to start them on a magnesium drip. Yet foods with plenty of magnesium never seem to get onto the list of things to consume for heart disease patients because doctors simply are not taught to think in terms of *preventative health*.

For minerals to be easily absorbed by the body, they must be chelated. However, bio or naturally chelated minerals are only found in raw foods such as *Spirulina* and *Chlorella*. Thus, they are vastly superior to processed minerals because of the enzyme potential and bio-available vitamins and minerals they possess.

Vitamins

Vitamins are known as cofactors in biochemistry because they work with minerals and enzymes and are worthless by themselves. Vitamins will also not function unless the right minerals in a balanced state are present in the body. This is why many vitamin supplements are nutritionally worthless. Vitamin and mineral supplements are amalgams of extracts and concentrates that may seem worthwhile in theory, but in practice simply don't work very well. Most make for some very expensive urine.

Whole Foods vs. Extracts and Concentrates

A common approach to fitness and health is to provide the body with supplements that will build particular parts of the body that a person wants to emphasize such as muscle definition. This is particularly true in sports training.

Bodybuilding is a perfect example where substances such as Creatin have gained a foothold. Creatin is a natural compound, which is used to supply energy to our muscles. It is produced in the liver, pancreas, and kidneys, and is used throughout the body's muscle tissue. Once it reaches the muscles, it is converted into phosphocreatine (creatine phosphate), a metabolite, which is used to regenerate the muscles' energy source, ATP (adenosine triphosphate). Results such as increased muscle mass can be dramatic when using creatin. Although completely natural when created by the body, consuming large amounts of creatin can cause serious imbalances in the body because it simply was not designed to work this way. Taking large amounts of any single vitamin such as Niacin can throw the whole body out of metabolic and hormonal balance.

It is quite unusual to become overstuffed or even sick from eating fresh fruits and vegetables whereas over-eating cooked foods is quite common. Fresh fruits and vegetables are never toxic. However, when taking extracts and concentrates, there is an inherent danger it will build up in the body and become toxic, even if they are naturally derived.

Fat

Foods fall into one of three categories: Fats, Carbohydrates and Proteins. What kind of fat you eat will substantially affect your overall health profile. Saturated fat is found primarily in animal fat and is harmful to the body, leading to cancer and other chronic diseases. It also clogs the arteries and dims mental faculties.

Essential fatty acids are required by the body and are found in abundance in the vegetable kingdom in foods such as avocado, sesame oil, olive oil, flaxseed oil, black and wild rice, almonds, hazelnuts, *Spirulina* and *Chlorella*. These are monounsaturated fats with antioxidant qualities that fend off arterial damage from LDL cholesterol. Other fatty acids such as Omega 3 and Omega 6 groups are found in certain kinds of fish such as trout, shark, crab, lobster and shrimp. However, only the Omega 6 group is healthy for the body. Essential fatty acids aid in the production of bodily and cellular messengers as well as other communication vehicles. Research has demonstrated that eating fat of any kind starts a chemical chain reaction of unparalleled and exquisite complexity in the cells themselves.

Fats offer tremendous benefits to the body. Whether the body is able to fight disease is often determined by fatty acids. However, assimilating and utilizing fats and fatty acids requires the presence of certain enzymes. Fat pharmacology, the study of fat and the human body, has incredible possibilities for curing and preventing disease.

Never cook or eat anything with canola oil in it. Canola oil (*Canadian oil*) is made from the rapeseed, which is quite bad for the body, especially digestion. It coats food and does not allow nutrients to be absorbed by the body because canola oil cannot itself be digested. In many countries, rapeseed oil is not even designated a food fit for human or animal consumption. Canola or rapeseed oil is used prevalently in processed foods. Virtually all commercial brand name peanut butters use rapeseed oil, not to mention they add sugar. At that point, the peanut butter and jelly sandwich you give your child has been robbed of much of its nutritional potential.

Carbohydrates

Carbohydrates are the fuel of the human body. There are simple, complex and starchy carbohydrates. Our body transforms starchy carbohydrates such as rice and potatoes into complex sugars that our body uses as fuel. It takes the body 18-24 hours to process starchy carbohydrates.

Simple carbohydrates such as fresh fruit are comprised of complex organic sugars that the body can use immediately upon consuming, which is why bananas are such a high energy food.

Protein must be consumed with carbohydrates in order for it to be effectively processed by the body. Not consuming carbohydrates with protein can lead to sudden weight gain because the carbohydrates are turned into fat by the body instead of sugar. Diets that remove or severely limit carbohydrates should be avoided since this can cause serious imbalances in the body and sudden weight gain for the same reason, carbohydrates being turned into fat by the body instead of sugar. Removing carbohydrates from your diet will cause sudden weight loss. However, when they are reintroduced, the body reacts in a way that causes sudden weight gain, often adding more pounds to the body than were taken off to begin with. Neither scenario is particularly healthy.

Proteins (*Amino Acids*)

Proteins are long complex chains of amino acids. They are the building blocks of our cells. Life would not be possible without them. Without amino acids, we cannot take nutrients into our body, especially when they are eaten raw with their enzymes intact. A wide array of amino acids are found in both *Spirulina* and *Chlorella,* more than any other whole food. Animal protein, or meat, is a difficult and exhausting way for the body to get amino acids. Meat, fish and eggs are pre-formed amino acids already constructed into the proteins that the animal's DNA has programmed or formed it into. The body must break down these pre-formed proteins into basic amino acids then reform them into the proteins that the human body needs. This uses energy and deposits acid waste in the bloodstream, which must then be discarded. It also adds to the overall acidic profile of the body.

Even though they are 60% protein, *Spirulina* and *Chlorella* produce a net alkaline effect in the body. Since their amino acids are not pre-formed proteins, it takes considerably less energy to assimilate them, which also creates less acid in the process.

Chapter 4

Raw (*Living*) Foods & Enzymes

Clearly, some time ago makers and consumers of American junk food passed jointly through some kind of sensibility barrier in the endless quest for new taste sensations. Now they are a little like those desperate junkies who have tried every known drug and are finally reduced to mainlining toilet bowl cleanser in an effort to get still higher.

~ Bill Bryson, *Journalist*

People naturally have an obsession with their food tasting good. Unfortunately, this often comes with a high price. Fat makes food taste good. Take half the fat out of cheddar cheese and you lose half the taste. We buy fast food at popular burger chains because the food is tasty, yet it is nothing more than a filler, a mechanism that flips the body's hunger switch off. Never mind that the meal has essentially no nutritional value, nor fiber.

There are foods that lead to life and foods that lead to death. Raw foods lead to life because they are themselves essentially alive, teaming with enzymes that make its nutrients immediately available to the body. Cooked, processed and pasteurized foods lead to death because they no longer contain the enzymes that make its nutrients bioavailable. Thus, cooked food has been changed from life renewing foods into mere sustenance that only provides the body with the nutrients it needs to get through the next hour, day, week or month. Cooked foods do not rejuvenate the body and its cells. Rather, they assist in the body's agonizingly slow demise, a silent accomplice never suspected for the large role it plays in disease and aging.

The first species of humanity to reveal chronic disease such as arthritis through fossil evidence was Neanderthal Man, the first species known to cook its food. The frigid environment in which they lived likely had nothing to do with the promulgation of chronic disease because if it did, then primitive Eskimos would also reveal they had similar diseases through fossil evidence, but there is none.

Enzymes are one of many numerous proteins or conjugated proteins produced by living organisms and functioning as biochemical catalysts.

Enzymes make life itself possible. Enzymes and enzyme reactions essentially are the fountain of life itself. They are required for every chemical reaction in the human body. We literally can't do anything without enzyme reactions: move, twitch, think, blink, walk, breath, talk, etc. Minerals, vitamins and hormones cannot function without the presence of enzymes. Even though every nutrient the body requires may be present, they are worthless to the body without *enzymes, the life force,* to make them function.

There are 100 trillion cells and millions of enzymes in the body. Every second, millions of cells die and are replaced by new cells that whose formation is caused by enzyme reactions. The human body forms millions of different proteins, enzymes and enzyme reactions that perform functions in every part of the body. Essentially they are what we are because they control all our physical and mental actions, reactions and movements. Smiling, for instance, is a complicated sequence of enzyme reactions. This demonstrates the divine complexity and genius of the human body.

Over 300 different enzyme reactions take place in the body every second. There are hundreds of thousands of enzymes in every organ, fluid and bodily tissue. We can use the analogy that the human body is a light bulb and enzymes are the electric currents that light it. Enzyme depletion results in ulcers, constipation, arthritis, PMS, chronic fatigue and a litany of other ailments and chronic diseases.

There are three enzyme sources for the body. Food enzymes are the external source and are derived exclusively from consuming raw fruits and vegetables. The body itself produces digestive and metabolic enzymes.

Metabolic enzymes are responsible for the growth of new cells, organ and tissue maintenance, each of which has its own specific enzyme group to do its work.

Enzymes are not true catalysts because catalysts are inorganic and do not contain energy within them the way enzymes do. Enzymes are charged with energy which is why they cannot be synthesized the way vitamins and minerals can. Enzymes emit a form of radiation as they react with other substances while performing their functions. Catalysts do not emit energy of any kind.

We can view enzymes in the human body as a kind of bank account. We constantly make withdrawals from the account as we use these enzymes, metabolic and digestive, especially when we eat cooked foods. More enzymes must constantly replace these enzymes or the bank account will be depleted. Deposits in the account are raw foods. Withdrawals are cooked foods. When we eat cooked foods we strain the digestive enzyme supply. Our bodies are born with the ability to produce a certain amount of enzymes and when our enzyme bank account runs dry and we have spent our congenital supply without replacing them, we take the first of many steps toward aging, disease, and eventually death. Once the body has been completely exhausted of its ability to produce certain enzymes, its organs begin to malfunction and the body quickly dies. Enzymes are one of the most critical pieces of the Great Health puzzle. The loss of the body's ability to produce enzymes is postulated by some to be the root cause of many degenerative diseases and undoubtedly this is true.

Civilization has revolved around a cooked food diet, one mostly void of enzymes, for thousands of years. Today's typical diet is so laden with cooked foods that the body is constantly overburdened with the difficulty of digesting that food because it has no enzymes. The consequence is that other areas of the body are robbed of their enzymes in order to meet the enzyme demands of digestion. The depletion of certain metabolic enzymes happens because the body is busy producing digestive enzymes, which are given top priority because it is paramount that more nutrients be constantly supplied to the body in great numbers, especially as we age.

Garlic, for instance, repeats on many people for hours after eating it. The reason is because it has been cooked , making it difficult for the body to digest and absorb its nutrients. Cooked foods are sometimes surrounded by oil, which makes digesting them even more difficult. This will not occur with raw garlic because its enzymes are intact, and therefore, the body readily assimilates it.

"It is interesting to note that when captive wild animals are fed a diet resembling human food in the sense of it being largely heat-treated, they develop diseases similar or identical to those found in human beings." [21]

Chronic disease, such as those found in humans, are virtually nonexistent in the wild, which is telling evidence to the detriment that an overly cooked food diet has on the body.

We are a society obsessed with the taste of our food, regardless of whether it has any nutritional value or not. Food is seen as a tasty filler. Nutritional value is given a back seat to taste and often is not considered at all.

People believe a low fat, high fiber, high quality diet is superior, which is true. Regardless, any diet that is not supplemented with water and raw foods, is seriously impaired. Ideally, 45-70% of our overall diet should be comprised of raw fruits and vegetables.

The Therapeutic Power of Sprouts

Spouts are cultured from the seeds or beans of any edible plant. They are extremely easy to grow and without doubt one of the most powerful whole foods we can consume. They are considered one of the only true living foods because they are actually growing when they are consumed.

Fruits and vegetables such as egg plant, broccoli or apples have stopped growing by the time they are consumed. They are the end product of a plant. Sprouts are the beginning of a plant. This difference is significant because the substances that are present in a plant when it has just sprouted are often not the same after it has flowered and produced fruit. In mature plants, these substances are often either no longer available or are present in greatly diminished quantities.

Sprouts are most valuable because of their ability to produce enzymes in huge quantities that cannot be found at any other point in that plant's growing process. Take broccoli sprouts for instance. Within three to five days of sprouting, they produce an enzyme called *sulforaphane* in quantities 40 to 50 times greater than that found in an entire head of mature broccoli. *Sulforaphane* is an extremely powerful cancer-fighting agent. Once this discovery was published at John Hopkins University in 1998, it wasn't long before supermarkets across the country were carrying broccoli sprouts.

Many bird species store seeds in a pouch or *crop* above their stomach for 10-14 hours while they take on moisture and begin to sprout. This is a clever way nature devised to provide enzymes to birds. There is a subtle, yet profound nutritional importance in this instinctual animal behavior.

How to Grow Sprouts

Although it is not necessary, sprouting equipment can be purchased at health food stores and on the Internet. It takes about 3-5 days for most seeds to properly sprout depending on the type. Beans generally take longer to sprout than seeds.

Start by soaking the seeds or beans in water, preferably Alkaline *Ionized Water,* for 12-18 hours then drain off the water so they remain moist, but are not soaking in the water where they can rot. Place a damp cloth or paper towel over the seeds to keep them from quickly drying out. They must remain moist at all times or they will not sprout. Rinse the sprouts about every 8-12 hours with cold water. This helps keep them moist and fresh by removing the bacteria that surrounds them. If you do not rinse them, the sprouts will become moldy and take on a musty smell.

Once the seeds have sufficiently sprouted, place them in sunlight for 8-12 hours. Only sprouted seeds should be put in sunlight. They will take on a greenish hue as they begin to produce chlorophyll, one of most important nutrients the body requires.

When sprouting beans of any kind, they do not need to be put in sunlight and can be consumed immediately after sprouting.

Fresh Herbs

Chew on raw oregano leaves and it will be an experience you will not soon forget because oregano sets one's mouth on fire as readily as hot peppers do. It's strong because of the density of the enzymes it contains. Herbs have healing properties and anything that can heal will be much more effective as a *preventative health* measure when consumed raw. People complain that one must consume such large amounts of herbs for them to be effective in healing the body. However, not as much is required when they are used in a *preventative health* fashion to deter disease from surfacing. And when eaten fresh, the enzymes make the herbs alive and thus require much smaller dosages for them to be effective.

Lettuce vs. Green Food

Lettuce is a very poor food. There is very little nutritional value in any of the varieties and most are low in fiber as well. Iceberg lettuce, ironically the most widely available, does little but pass through the body because it contains a substance that prevents the stomach from actually digesting it.

Spinach and other greens such as beet leaves, sprouts, parsley and kale contain vastly higher nutritional value than lettuce. Look for vegetable greens that are dense and possess purple or red hues because they contain the strongest cleansing and antioxidant qualities found in nature. Another substitute for a salad base are sprout greens such as sunflower or buckwheat sprouts. They are powerful foods compared to lettuce simply because they are packed with enzymes found only in the earliest stages of a plant's evolution. They are also far more flavorful than lettuce.

Olive Oil

Ancient Greeks and Romans considered olive oil a staple of their diet. Olive oil is an extraordinary food that should be consumed by everyone. It can be used in place of butter and in every aspect of cooking. Cold pressed extra virgin olive oil is the best, but because of its extraordinary health benefits, any grade of olive oil is better than most other oils.

Other healthy oils are grape seed, flax and sesame oil. The fat found in these oils help lower cholesterol. The presence of fat in the diet is extremely important. A very low fat diet can actually raise LDL (bad) cholesterol and lower HDL (good) cholesterol levels, the exact opposite of what we need.

Butter is mostly useless fat. It is high in bad cholesterol, as is all animal fat. Even though it is a dairy product, butter is superior to margarine, which should be completely avoided. Margarine is full of unwanted synthetic substances and trans fatty acids (found in all meat and dairy products), which have been shown to be quite harmful.

In Search of Great Digestion

Having great digestion after every meal is the only way to live. I mean that literally and figuratively. Living with chronic stomach problems is a prison term that people condemn *themselves* to: stomach acid, acid reflux syndrome, gas, nausea, etc. We can have the best digestion imaginable if we just follow a few simple rules.

Don't drink water 30 minutes before a meal, during and at lest 30 minutes after a meal. Drinking water or other liquids dilutes the digestive process by washing out bacteria, hydrochloric acid (HCL) and enzymes that are required for proper digestion. Consume a lot of water 30 minutes before eating. About 15 minutes before the meal, take a supplement containing the two *friendly bacteria* the body needs: *Lactobacillus* Acidophilus and Bifidus. These are known as intestinal floral. Each performs a different function in a different part of the digestive tract. By taking them before a meal, we are priming the digestive tract to receive food so its nutrients can be efficiently extracted, and used by the body.

Without the friendly bacteria in our systems, our health is in jeopardy for several reasons. Without them, the body cannot properly assimilate nutrients and keep the digestive wall clean, which is critical to well being. Urinary tract infections brought on by *Candida* and other yeast infections women experience can often be remedied by consuming these bacteria. They are especially useful when taken with *Chlorella* because it causes these bacteria to multiply at four times the normal rate. Ironically, doctors often prescribe antibiotics to treat urinary tract infections, which kill off these friendly bacteria.

The lack of these friendly bacteria provides an opportunity for harmful bacteria that are parasitic in nature to get a foothold in the digestive tract. Bacteria cause stomach ulcers. This can lead to a host of problems as well as aggravate some existing ones. Obviously we want to avoid any bacteria from flourishing in us except those our digestive tract requires. This can be achieved by providing the body with these friendly bacteria on a regular basis, at least 2-3 times a week, if not daily.

After taking the bacteria with 3-4 grams of *Chlorella,* the next thing that should be consumed is *Spirulina* and other raw foods, a salad for instance. This further prepares the upper stomach to properly extract nutrients from the food we send it, regardless of whether it is raw or cooked.

Chewing causes the mouth to produce saliva and the stomach to produce HCL. Saliva contains an enzyme, *amylase*, which begins the conversion of starch (carbohydrates) into simple sugars. Along with enzymes, HCL breaks down the amino acids and other substances in the food so the body can assimilate the nutrients. We do not want to consume any liquids that will dilute or wash away these digestive substances such as bacteria, HCL and our digestive enzymes.

Ginger root is also a superior digestive aide. Ginger is unique amongst foods. Like any other food, eating ginger in its raw form is the best way to get the most nutritional benefit from it. The enzymes help the ginger to assimilate quickly and effectively, providing additional nutrients to the body that would not be found in the food if it were cooked. Digestion is significantly enhanced by the intake of ginger before and even after a meal. Try mincing 2 to 3 grams of raw ginger and taking it before a meal with the *Chlorella.* Ginger is an extremely strong, spicy food, which is an indication of its nutritional strength. Ginger is also a powerful immune system builder.

The quest for Great Digestion is nothing new unless it's viewed on an evolutionary scale. Poor digestion came with the advent of man cooking his food. People complain about stomach acid after a meal more than any other digestion ailment. If the condition is bad enough, it occurs even between meals. Heartburn is a warning signal from the body's digestive system. It is informing us that whatever it is we are putting in our body, it's not the right kind of food and too much of it is cooked. Heartburn comes from eating acid foods, junk foods, processed and fast foods, drinking soft drinks or alcohol and *from not eating raw foods with a meal.* In fact, removing raw fruits and vegetables from the diet will eventually insure digestive problems of one sort or another.

One of the most insidious digestive-aide products to come on the market is the stomach-acid blocker, which allows people to eat whatever they please without the worry of heartburn. What's worse is that doctors regularly prescribe them. If there has ever been a product that hides the symptoms of potentially serious gastral problems, it is digestive stomach-acid blockers. They should be avoided at all times. If you have chronic stomach acid problems, your body is screaming at you to stop the endless onslaught of harmful, indigestible cooked foods that are void of nutrition, especially enzymes.

Organic vs. Inorganic

Unfortunately, most foods we find in supermarkets today are contaminated with pesticides, herbicides and other chemical additives. While growing crops in this manner allows for volume production, these chemicals undeniably end up in whomever consumes them.

However, finding good quality certified organic fruits and vegetables at a reasonable price can be difficult. Organic is definitely better. Compare what is grown in a summer garden to what is bought in the store. The difference in look and quality is often quite dramatic.

The question remains whether to eat foods that are grown using pesticides, herbicides and chemical fertilizers. In many cases, we do not have a choice because quality organic foods are not readily available. Even though all raw foods have detoxification properties, when you consume foods that come with chemical substances that are foreign to the body, they work against us.

It is impossible to completely get away from naturally occurring pollutants such as heavy metals, which are replete throughout our environment. Commercially grown foods are better than cooked foods any day. However, if you can find it and afford it, organic is well worth the money.

How Often We Should Eat

Gluttony is an emotional escape, a sign something is eating us.

~ Peter De Vries

Lunch is for wimps.

~ Oliver Stone

Even though I don't think he meant it this way, Oliver Stone is right. We should eat moderate size meals several hours apart. In general, people eat far too often during the day. After eating, we should wait at least 30 minutes to one hour for our meal to digest, then purge our systems by drinking as much water as possible. It takes our bodies several hours to fully digest a meal, but some water should be consumed during this time because the digestive process requires a great deal of water.

Upon waking in the morning, our primary goal should be to rehydrate the body after the drought of not drinking any liquids in the last 6 to 9 hours. Unfortunately, many people reach for dehydrating substances such as coffee or soft drinks, in many cases strictly for the caffeine. These are the last substances anyone ought to consume after waking in the morning. A glass of strong *Ionized Water* will wake you up naturally and every bit as well as caffeinated beverages. It provides oxygen and rehydrates the body, both of which are quite energizing.

Daily purging of the digestive tract with water, especially *Ionized Water*, is essential for digestive health.

You will be amazed at how much energy, vigor and mental sharpness you will have throughout the day if you start by drinking sufficient amounts of *Ionized Water* and eating *Chlorella, Spirulina,* raw fruits and vegetables. They provide a solid nutritional foundation that can be built on throughout the day and do not require much energy to be digested.

A light lunch, or no lunch at all, will not tax the body's energy reserve with the need for digestion. Carbohydrates such as bread, rice and potatoes should be avoided during the day because they require a great deal of energy to digest and often work as an afternoon soporific that makes us drowsy. Carbohydrates are best consumed primarily in the evenings because their drain on the body's energy reserves helps provide us with a good night's sleep.

Dietary Fiber

One of the biggest pieces of the overall health picture that is missing from many people lives is dietary fiber. Most of us make little or no attempt to be certain that an adequate amount of fiber is present in our diet, yet dietary fiber is what cleans out our digestive system and helps keep it healthy.

When cattle ranchers removed dietary fiber (hay) from their steer's diet and fed them only grain in order to sooner ready them for the market, the result was that *e-coli (escherichia coli bacterium)* surfaced in the meat, a parasitic and extremely dangerous bacteria that can be deadly. The same happens to humans who remove dietary fiber from their diet. Fiber cleans the inner lining of the digestive tract so it can take in nutrients and excrete digestive juices. Without dietary fiber, neither of these activities can take place because of blockages. Thus it allows parasitic bacteria to thrive in place of the friendly bacteria.

A diet void of fiber will lead to digestive diseases of all kinds, intestinal blockages, hemorrhoids, even colon cancer, especially when combined with an acidic diet and substances such as soft drinks and hard liquor.

Chlorella is especially high in dietary fiber, as are a host of other fruits and vegetables, especially if they are raw and the dietary fiber has not lost some of its effectiveness to cooking. Bananas are a great source of dietary fiber, as is pineapple. This is especially true of the pineapple core where the highest concentration of *bromalain* is found, which is an essential digestive enzyme.

The Myth of Meat

Meat is the center of the Western diet. Meat is one of the most popular foods in the world. In countries where it is not the center of the diet, such as in India, it is usually because those countries do not have the resources to efficiently raise, slaughter and store meat. It is not because they don't want to eat it.

We are taught from an early age that meat is the best food we can eat. Meat, in reality, is an inferior food. It is an extraordinary chore for the body to digest meat compared to *Spirulina*, *Chlorella* and other raw fruits and vegetables. Since meat contains **no** dietary fiber, it requires a lot of fiber from other sources in order to be properly digested, otherwise it hangs up in the digestive system for days, sometimes longer, and becomes a drag on the entire body, robbing it of resources and energy.

The protein found in meat must be broken down into amino acids so they can be reformed into the protein chains that the human body requires. *Spirulina* and *Chlorella* are composed of amino acids that are immediately ready to be formed into complex proteins. These amino acids are considered pre-digested protein, unlike meat that is not. Cooked meat does not contain enzymes, unlike raw foods that are self-digestible.

Meat contains only 11 amino acids compared with the 18 amino acids contained in *Spirulina* and *Chlorella*. Meat is not a complete protein while *Spirulina* and *Chlorella* are.

Protein, which is comprised of *amino acids,* is by its very nature acidic. The difficult digestibility and high fat content of meat also contributes to the high amounts of acid meat releases into the body. New techniques to make meat more tender repeatedly apply an electric current to the carcass. This releases natural acids into the meat, which tenderizes it, yet unfortunately makes the meat even more acidic to the body.

Although the body requires essential fatty acids from vegetables, the body cannot use animal fat. It becomes a complete waste product for the body, adding to its overall acidity.

Cattle are given numerous antibiotics, steroids and other pharmaceuticals that end up in the meat people consume. Needless to say these substances are not healthy for us. Consuming meat that contains residual antibiotics interferes with digestion by destroying the friendly bacteria in the stomach. Meat that contains animal steroids inhibits the natural balance of the human body, as will animal hormones. This is especially true of children who depend on correct hormone levels to grow properly. Whenever possible, choose meat that has been raised organically, i.e., without the use of animal steroids, hormones and high levels of antibiotics.

Vegetarians often do not get enough vitamin B-12, which is found in meat. A deficiency in vitamin B-12 can lead to blindness. *Spirulina* and *Chlorella* are extremely high in the entire vitamin B complex, which is synonymous with high energy. B vitamins are somewhat ineffective if they are not all consumed together. For example, take the practice of giving vitamin B-12 shots to those suffering from anemia. Although this may be of some limited help in the short term, it is not nearly as effective as eating a whole food that contains the entire vitamin B complex.

Meat is eaten for taste and as a stomach filler, nothing more. By stomach filler, I mean it is a food that stays in the digestive tract for many hours because it is so difficult to digest. Although it may keep a person from getting too hungry in the middle of the afternoon when dinner is still hours away, a slow digestive system works against the body in many ways. The quicker foods are digested, have their nutrients removed and exit the body, the better.

Meat is a maintenance food. It sustains and keeps the body functioning, but it certainly does not renew nor provide it with the plethora of vitamins, minerals, amino acids, carbohydrates and enzymes that foods such as *Spirulina* and *Chlorella* possess.

Acid Forming Foods, Drinks and Activities

Smoking, hard liquor, legal and illicit drugs and soft drinks are the most destructive substances a person can put in their body. What they have in common more than anything else is that they are extremely acidic. Although one or more of the chemically addictive substances founds in today's cigarette may cause cancer and other disease, it's the acid residue of the smoke itself that prepares the perfect environment for disease to flourish in the body.

Everyone falls victim to stress in their daily lives. It is the nature of life itself to be exposed to stressful situations. Stress can cause chemical and hormonal changes in the body that disrupt its delicate balance. In some people, it can lead to headaches, muscle tension, sleep disturbance, high blood pressure, cardiovascular disease and a host of other ailments. It produces free radicals in the body, which lead to cellular deterioration and premature aging. Stress also produces large amounts of acid in the body, which leads to digestive problems and further deterioration of its cells, organs and tissue. The acid produced from stress is an extremely harmful byproduct to the human body.

The Danger of Soft Drinks

Soft drinks disturb the calcium/phosphorous ratio balance by leaching these alkaline minerals to balance their extreme acidic state. The sugar in soft drinks leaches the mineral ions from the body eventually depleting them. It erodes the teeth the way the ocean erodes a sandy beach. Don't be fooled, diet drinks are no better. The aspartame in diet soft drinks has been solidly linked to liver damage. The word *soda* comes from the excessive amount of sodium soft drinks contain. Soft drinks are laden with phosphoric acid and sodium, which destroy the nephrons, or filters, of the kidneys. They also contain high levels of aluminum ions from the cans they are packaged in.

The negative health effects of consuming soft drinks are slow to surface, sometimes taking years to manifest themselves. However, there are instances of chronic pop drinkers who contract osteoporosis in their thirties. The condition occurs because the calcium in the bones is overused as a buffering agent to counteract the extreme acidity of the soft drinks. To put the damage that soft drinks do to the body into proper perspective, it takes 20-25 glasses of Alkaline *Ionized Water* to negate the resulting acid effect on the body of one soft drink.

While hard drugs such as heroin and cocaine will destroy the mind, their effect on the body is not nearly as detrimental as soft drinks. Soft drinks are truly at the top of the list of horrible things we put in our bodies.

Top Ten Reasons We Should Never Consume Soft Drinks!

1. Soft drinks steal water from the body in order to process their high levels of sugar. They work very much like a diuretic that takes away more water than it provides to the body. To replace the water stolen and negate the acid effects of soft drinks, a person needs to drink 20-25 glasses of *Ionized Water* for every one soft drink!
2. Soft drinks never quench your thirst, and certainly not your body's need for water. Constantly denying your body adequate amounts of water will lead to *Chronic Cellular Dehydration,* a condition that weakens the body at the cellular level. This, in turn, will lead to a weakened immune system and a plethora of diseases.
3. The elevated levels of phosphates in soft drinks leach vital minerals from the body. Soft drinks are made with purified water that also leach minerals from the body. A severe lack of minerals can lead to heart disease (lack of magnesium), osteoporosis (lack of calcium), mental disease (lack of phosphorous), as well as many other diseases. Vitamins cannot perform their function in the body without the presence of these and other alkaline minerals.
4. Soft drinks can remove rust from a car bumper or other metal surfaces. Imagine what it's doing to your digestive tract, as well as the rest of your body.

5. The high amounts of sugar in soft drinks causes the pancreas to produce an abundance of insulin, which leads to a "sugar crash". Chronic elevation and depletion of sugar and insulin can lead to diabetes and other imbalance-related diseases. This is particularly disruptive to growing children for whom soft drink consumption can lead to life-long health problems.
6. Soft drinks severely interfere with digestion. Caffeine and high amounts of sugar virtually shut down the digestive process. That means the body is essentially taking in NO nutrients from any food just eaten. When consumed with french fries and other fried foods, which can take weeks to digest, there is arguably nothing worse a person can put in their body short of actual poison. The typical burger and fries fast food meal is a kind of slow death in a sack.
7. Diet soft drinks contain aspartame, which has been solidly linked to depression, insomnia, neurological disorder, liver disease and a plethora of other diseases. The FDA has received more than 10,000 consumer complaints about aspartame, that's 80% of all complaints about food additives, more than any other on record.
8. Soft Drinks are EXTREMELY acidic, so much so that they sometimes eat through the liner of an aluminum can and leach aluminum ions from it. Alzheimer patients who have been autopsied often have high levels of aluminum in their brains. Heavy metals in the body can lead to many neurological and other diseases.
9. Soft drinks are EXTREMELY acidic: The human body prefers a pH of about 7.0. Soft drinks have a pH of 2.5. Since the pH scale is logarithmic, this means that soft drinks are literally 100,000's of times more acidic than the body! Diseases flourish in an acidic environment. If not for the miracle of homeostasis, the acid alone in soft drinks would kill us instantly. Homeostasis is the body's ability to quickly compensate from the influx of acid and alkaline substances that are ingested. Soft drinks deposit large amounts of acid waste in the body, which accumulate in the joints, between the cells, and around the organs.
10. Soft drinks are the WORST THING you can possibly put in your body, especially when you are sick. Consuming soft drinks when you are ill with a cold, flu or something worse will only make it that much harder for the body to fight the disease.

"Soft drink consumption in industrial societies is epidemic and the problems that spring from it are as serious as the effects of alcohol usage . . . The list of diseases related to soft drink consumption is staggering, but reversible." [22]

Processed foods

I can think of nothing worse than a fast food burger meal of substandard meat, white bread, french fries and a soft drink. I ate my share of them before I learned how horrible they truly are for your health. Neither the meat, french fries nor white bread has any dietary fiber. *Strike One.* If you skin potatoes, slice them thin to expose their surface area, freeze then deep fry them in oil, there is no fiber, nutrition, minerals, nothing left but a wad of acidic starchy waste that is impossible to digest. It can take *weeks* for them to move through the digestive system. *Strike Two.* The caffeine and acid level of soft drinks shuts down the digestive system precluding the possibility that the body might actually absorb any nutrients. *Strike Three.* After having spent the money, you're less healthy and more acidic than when you started. *Bon Appetite!*

Any food that has been processed has had most of its nutritional value removed. Processed foods need to be *enriched* because they have been robbed of all their nutrients so what remains is something resembling food grade cardboard. Naturally, the nutrients that have been removed must now be replaced. The feeble attempts to replace them with synthetic vitamins and other man-made nutrients are pathetic and will not be effectively absorbed and utilized by the body. Processed foods are packed with chemical preservatives and other alien substances that when consumed, have unknown effects on the body and its delicate chemistry. They do little more than help create an overly acidic condition in the body.

A regular diet of potato chips, corn chips, massed produced cookies, fruit rolls, candy and cake snacks packed with processed sugar and other elements has helped an entire generation of children to have the highest cancer rates in history, and allowed what were traditionally adult diseases such as diabetes to become commonplace as childhood diseases.

The biggest problem with processed foods is that they are void of *enzymes*. Eating foods that are cooked, pasteurized or otherwise processed puts a tremendous strain on the body's enzyme supply and the ability to digest those foods. The rise of processed foods beginning in the 1930's and the rise of cancer rates during that same period illustrates the startling correlation between the two. The advent of processed foods was the beginning of the systematic removal of freshness from our diet, which helped end the habit of eating raw fruits and vegetables. History will one day show what a great health calamity the advent of processed food truly was.

Fried Foods

It's very difficult for the body to absorb the nutrients from any food that is covered in oil or animal fat. French fries are a prime example of a food, the potato, which has been completely robbed of any nutritional benefit. The potato should be cooked with its peel, the most alkaline part of a potato that provides it with balance so it does not create acidity in the body.

Fried foods allow vital nutrients to pass through the body instead of being absorbed by it. They also lead to higher cholesterol and coronary heart disease.

All fried foods create enormous amounts of acid in the body. It causes the digestive tract to slow and become clogged. It coats the inner lining of the digestive tract so the body cannot absorb nutrients. This becomes a breeding ground for molds, fungi, viruses, bacteria and disease in general. Combined with a low fiber diet, it is the reason why colon cancer is one of the most common forms of cancer.

Chocolate

Chocolate happens to be one of my favorites of all time; however, it should be avoided. It is extremely toxic to the body, has quite of lot of caffeine and is produced using processed sugar. Chocolate is also very bad for digestion and should never be consumed directly after a meal.

Authors speak of the great value of foods such as ginger root, shataki mushrooms and garlic, then encourage people to have luxurious chocolate deserts as a reward. This kind of *sin on Saturday and repent on Sunday* mentality serves to demonstrate how little knowledge such authors actually possess about nutrition and proper digestion. Sweets should be avoided immediately after dinner, especially chocolate because it can impair the digestive process by introducing too much sugar into the body too quickly. I wait one to two hours after mealtime before having a sweet desert.

One positive thing to report about chocolate is that, surprisingly, it does have some antioxidant properties, as does coffee. Coffee is a diuretic that should be avoided, especially in the morning because caffeine virtually shuts down the digestive system.

Dairy Products

Removing dairy products from your diet can be of profound benefit to your overall health. Dairy products create mucous in the body, especially if they have been pasteurized, which virtually all are. Dairy operations often inject steroids, hormones and other pharmaceuticals into the cows they raise, which of course ends up in the milk we drink, having a negative effect on the body as it mixes with its chemistry.

I was once a great lover of dairy products of all kinds, but once I removed them from my diet, I immediately noticed a tremendous difference in my health. It took about three months to completely get the *dairy* and its related mucous out of my system. My sinus problems decreased significantly. I no longer had a stuffy nose 300 days out of the year. My skin pores felt cleaner and skin blemishes diminished in number. I no longer experienced chest congestion or phlegm, especially after eating.

I have suffered from allergies two times a year since childhood. For three weeks of every summer I would be nearly incapacitated by tree pollen allergies and for three weeks in the fall I would be miserable with ragweed allergies. Once I removed dairy products from my diet, I experienced only minor allergy symptoms in June and almost none in the fall. It was an amazing reversal. I cured myself of an ailment I'd had since I was a child simply by removing a harmful food group.

Why dairy products produce so much mucous is obvious. They are viscous and mucous-like by their very nature. When milk was fed to dairy cattle, all the cattle became sick and/or died. This in itself demonstrates that we have no business consuming dairy products to begin with. Milk is meant for infants, which is why most animals and mammals produce it. Consuming it any other time in life is unhealthy, despite one of the longest marketing campaigns in history extolling the nutritional fortitude and purity of milk and other dairy products. Milk has the great advantage of being white, which makes it look like something that is naturally good for us.

Mucous causes a plethora of problems in people, especially allergies. And nothing creates more mucous in the body than dairy products. They cause congestion and labored breathing. Too much mucous will gum up the sinuses, throat, esophagus lungs and respiratory passages. Wheat products also create mucous in the body.

Neither should ever be consumed when you are sick, especially with a chronic disease.

The Danger of Aluminum

Aluminum is found is antiperspirants, not deodorants. It is commonly used in cooking pots and pans and is also found in many antacids, especially the liquid kind. Whether it's canned beer or soft drinks, stay clear of aluminum. *Chlorella* is the only natural substance known that binds with heavy metals such as aluminum, tin and mercury to effectively pull them out.

Chapter 5

Chlorella

(Chlorella Pyrenoidosa)

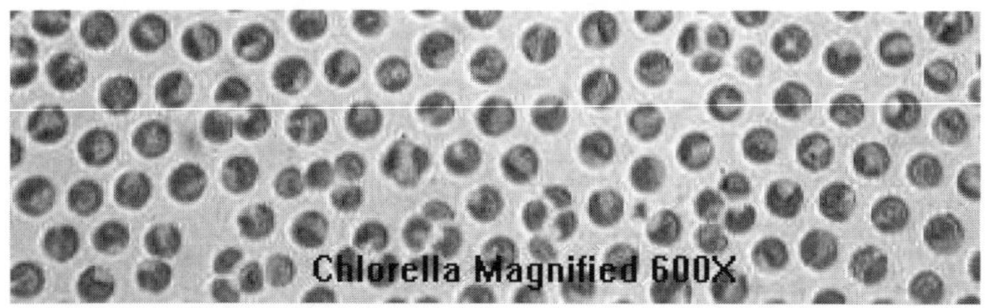
Chlorella Magnified 600X

The Most Magnificent Food in the World

"There is only one thing in the world worse than being talked about, and that is not being talked about."

~ Oscar Wilde
The Picture of Dorian Gray

Chlorella is not well known in the West. However, it ought to be talked about more than any other food because it is easily the most powerful food in the world. The *Chlorella* that is spoken of in this book is a very particular strain of algae known as *Chlorella Pyrenoidosa*. *Chlorella* is a single-celled plant that gets its name from the high amount of chlorophyll it contains. It is a green, fresh water micro-algae, one of the oldest foods on the planet. Fossils exist of *Chlorella Pyrenoidosa* that are over 2.5 billion years old. *Chlorella* contains the entire B complex, vitamins E & C and has a wide range of minerals, including magnesium, zinc, folic acid, phosphorous, potassium, iron and calcium. Anyone can take it regardless of their age, from a weaned infant to the elderly.

Chlorella is often referred to as *Broken Cell Chlorella* or *Cracked Cell Chlorella* because the outer cell wall is comprised of an indigestible fiber. So to get at the nutrients, the cell wall must be cracked or broken open.

There are two reliable methods for cracking *Chlorella's* cell wall. One is to crush the cell wall so the nutrients can be reached. However, there is a risk that the nutrients themselves can either be damaged or the cell wall not entirely broken open, only dented.

The other method of cracking *Chlorella's* cell wall is the use of pressure differential. This process builds pressure in a tank where the *Chlorella* is stored then suddenly released, causing the cell wall to gently rupture. This is the most organic, effective, safest and delicate method for breaking *Chlorella's* cell wall while still leaving the nutrients and enzymes intact.

Chlorella is one of the most scientifically studied foods in history. Numerous experiments have been run to determine exactly what substances are in *Chlorella* and it still is not exactly clear what some of them are. However, there is ample evidence that *Chlorella* stimulates tissue repair and overall growth like no other food known.

One of the things to take into account when considering the nutritional fortitude of a food is its age, more exactly, how long it has existed on the planet. For instance, fresh wheat grass is a strong food, full of enzymes and other nutrients. However, it has only existed for millions of years, which is negligible compared to the nearly 2.5 billion years *Chlorella* has existed. Therefore, wheat grass does not have anywhere near the broad spectrum of nutrients. The older the food, the more powerful and concentrated its nutrients tend to be.

Between *Spirulina* and *Chlorella*, *Chlorella* is definitely the more powerful of the two. While *Spirulina is* a powerful whole food, one of the strongest and purest in existence, *Chlorella* has properties that gives it a slight edge over *Spirulina.*

Chlorella takes inorganic chemicals and transforms them into active bio-available nutrients that have been directly formed and supercharged by sunlight. It can be grown virtually anywhere in the world as long as the climate is not too cold.

Powerful Nutraceutical

Chlorella is considered a *nutraceutical* because it provides the body with the proper nutrients it requires so it can heal itself. The human body is perfectly capable of healing itself if it is provided with the necessary vitamins, minerals, enzymes, amino acids and other nutrients its cells require. Nutraceuticals work to force the disease out of the body by building its cells and essentially leaving no room for disease to live.

"Chlorella is a wonderful food supplement and it will work best and most rapidly if combined with a correctly balanced and proportioned food regimen." [23]

There are many foods that have healing and preventative health qualities, but none possess such a powerful, wide-ranging and diverse group of nutrients as *Chlorella.* *"The minerals, vitamins, enzymes and amino acids that are contained in Chlorella supply all that the human system needs for good health."* [24]

Pharmaceuticals are designed to control disease by overcoming the body and destroying the disease. However, they always come with side effects and often only disguise the symptoms of the disease, never attacking its actual root cause and therefore often not curing the person. As a result, the body often doesn't rid itself of the disease, but simply puts it into remission.

Drugs are substances that are foreign to the body. Pharmaceuticals are not nutrients that naturally belong in the body, therefore they tend to have very immediate and dramatic effects on the body such as lowering blood pressure within days and sending migraine headaches away within hours. But if the root of the problem remains, what good are pharmaceuticals other than palliatives that provide temporary relief? Nutrients work to strengthen the body, pharmaceuticals fight for control over it.

"No medical claims are being made for Chlorella. I know that Chlorella is a food, not a medicine. We should realize, however, that when the proper foods are used, together with the right supplements to build up the health level of the body, diseases are often 'crowded out'. This is nature's way of healing the body. To put it very simply, there is no room for disease in a healthy body." [25]

Encourages Production of Interferon

Interferon is one of the body's best natural defenses against cancer. Interferon has been used for decades as a cancer treatment. T-cells in the body are active against viruses and cancer. Macrophages are large cells that surround and digest foreign substances in the body. They are active against cancer, foreign proteins and other chemicals. There are a finite number of macrophages in the human body, therefore limiting the ability of the body to remove harmful substances from the blood.

Chlorella has been shown to promote the production of macrophages and interferon. *"Interferon is a natural secretion of the body and is thought to be a physiological stimulator of macrophages.... Many more studies also demonstrate that Chlorella stimulates the immune system by way of macrophage stimulation."* [26]

One of the ways to fight cancer is the use of agents to stimulate macrophage production and activity. *Chlorella* stimulates the activity of T-cells and macrophages by increasing interferon levels thus enhancing the immune system's ability to combat foreign invaders whether they are bacteria, viruses, chemical substances, cancer cells or foreign proteins.

Chlorophyll and Magnesium Promote Cardiovascular Health

The name *Chlorella* derives from two Latin words *Chlor,* green leaf, referring to its unusually high content of chlorophyll, and *ella,* small, referring to the micro size of *Chlorella.* The chlorophyll gives *chlorella* its characteristic deep emerald-green color. *Chlorella* contains more chlorophyll than any other plant, 10 times that of *Spirulina,* which is itself considered high in chlorophyll.

Chlorophyll gives *Chlorella* its somewhat grassy taste and smell. Chlorophyll cells are nearly identical to hemoglobin (red blood cells) with one exception: Chlorophyll has a magnesium molecule at that center of it and hemoglobin has an iron molecule at the center of it. This is important because magnesium is essential for the heart to function properly. Every time our heart beats, magnesium is being utilized.

Chlorophyll has been used successfully in the treatment of cardiac hypertension. It is effective against anemia and stimulates the production of red blood cells in the body. It also helps carry oxygen around the body, especially to the brain. This is why *Chlorella* is often called *brain food*.

"The chlorophyll molecule is very similar to the hemoglobin molecule in blood, and it acts as a wonderful cleanser in the bowel, kidneys, liver and bloodstream. Green plants help build red blood cell count and control calcium in the body. Chlorella contains as high as 7% chlorophyll, 35 times more than we find in alfalfa." [27]

Contains Natural Digestive Enzymes
Aides Digestion, Bad Breath, Constipation

Chlorella contains large amounts of enzymes such as chlorophyllase and pepsin, which are digestive enzymes. Like *Spirulina*, *Chlorella* is packed with enzymes.

It only takes *Chlorella* one to three days to clear up a malfunctioning digestive tract. However, this does not mean that you should continue to consume junk food because *Chlorella* will compensate for it. This is the mistake people make when taking stomach acid blockers and then eating anything they want, even if is harmful to the body.

If someone has bad breath it is because their food is essentially rotting in their stomachs and not being properly digested. It is a sign that their digestive tract is stalled. There is no better food available than *Chlorella* to get a floundering digestive tract working properly again.

Chlorella reproduces at an incredible rate, quadrupling every 48 hours. It causes the beneficial bacteria in our stomach (*Lactobacillus Acidophilus)* to multiply at four times the normal rate. This greatly enhances digestion as well as the body's ability to absorb nutrients. *"Subsequent experiments with young animals and children showed that adding Chlorella to the diet caused increases in weight and size.*[28]

Chlorella is also extremely high in dietary fiber, which is crucial to digestive health. It is a unique fiber unlike any other and considered one of the best dietary fibers known.

Proper digestion is one of the keys to Great Health and there are few foods that provide such excellent digestion as *Chlorella*!

Best Known Natural Detoxifier of
Heavy Metals and other Synthetics

Chlorella's fibrous, indigestible outer shell is a dietary fiber that has been proven to actually bind with heavy metals and other synthetics that have accumulated in the body and pull them out. This fiber comprises approximately 20% of *Chlorella's* total cell mass.

"A Japanese study of heavy metal poisoning with cadmium revealed that when eight grams of Chlorella were administered to the test

animals daily, cadmium excretion increased threefold in the stool and sevenfold in the urine." [29]

The Japanese used *Chlorella* to significantly reduce radiation levels in exposed humans after the Hiroshima and Nagasaki atomic detonations.

"We can do experiments to show that Chlorella absorbs heavy metals from water. So if you use Chlorella as a nutritional supplement it will remove heavy metals such as lead, mercury and cadmium from the body." [30]

"Chlorella binds strongly to cadmium and will not give it up to the body. Dr. T. Nagano at Shizuoka College of Pharmacy in Japan did a study in which rats were given Chlorella that contained cadmium to determine whether the cadmium would be absorbed from the Chlorella into the rats. In rats given only cadmium (without Chlorella), growth retardation was noted, while no problem with growth was seen in those given Chlorella containing cadmium." [31]

Chlorella has been used to detoxify people suffering from PCB (polychlorobiphenyl) poisoning. It has also been used to treat chlordecone (kepone) toxicity, a harmful chlorinated hydrocarbon insecticide, and found to remove the chemical from the body more than twice as quickly than if treated without it. Dr. S. Pore of the West Virginia University School of Medicine found that mice were thoroughly detoxified from this toxin and that its half-life decreased from 40 days to 19 days.

"Clean blood efficiently carries off metabolic wastes from the cells and tissues. I believe the buildup of metabolic wastes in under-active body organs and systems is just as dangerous as an exposure to air and water pollution, nutritionally deficient foods and exposure to chemicals in the workplace." [32]

Chlorella will begin to significantly cleanse the blood and organs after a period of one to three months of consuming it, depending on the dosage taken. Consuming 15-25 grams of *Chlorella* per day is appropriate for someone trying to detoxify or combat a disease with the amazing cleansing properties of *Chlorella*. Since *Chlorella* is a whole food, not a concentrate or extract, you cannot take too much of it because of its detoxifying abilities. However, unlike pharmaceuticals, whole foods must be given time to rebuild the cells and the body so it can effectively fight disease.

"The cell wall itself has a beneficial effect. When Chlorella is used as a food, fragments of the cell wall adhere to and remove heavy metals like cadmium, lead and mercury from the body." [33]

"The detoxification capability of Chlorella is due to its unique cell wall and the material associated with it. Laboratory studies showed that there were two active absorbing substances - sporopollenin (a naturally occurring carotene like polymer which is resistant to degradation) and the algae cell walls." [34]

Helpful in the Fight against Alzheimer's, Dementia & Attention Deficit Disorder

Many elderly psychiatric patients have been shown to have high levels of heavy metals and other toxic substances concentrated in their brains. *Chlorella* binds with all heavy metals to remove them. To remove heavy metals and other toxins effectively will take 10 – 20 grams of *Chlorella* per day for several months before significant detoxification of these substances can be expected.

The enormous amount of chlorophyll in *Chlorella* provides oxygen to the brain, aiding with alertness and mental focus. Combined with the other blood-cleansing properties of *Chlorella*, it can be of great benefit to anyone suffering from various forms of mental deterioration. Chronic dehydration and improper diet certainly can lead to neurochemical imbalances of all kinds.

Powerful Immune System Builder: The Mysterious *Chlorella* Growth Factor (CGF)

Chlorella has the ability to quadruple every 20 hours, which no other plant or substance on Earth can do. It is programmed into *Chlorella's* DNA to do so; however, it is the CGF, Chlorella Growth Factor, that is actually responsible for this. This miraculous substance causes children and young animals to grow at a much faster rate than normal. In adults and children alike, it builds the immune system in ways no other food can.

"Chlorella contains 180 mg of beta-carotene in each 100 grams. Beta-carotene has the greatest vitamin A activity and antioxidant activity of all the known carotenoids... The immune system is as susceptible as any other system in the body to free radical damage... Extracts of algae were also studied and were shown to be more effective than beta-carotene alone." [35]

For example, a group of 100 Japanese sailors were exposed to the cold virus. Those who took two grams of *Chlorella* per day had 41% fewer colds than those who did not. Two grams of *Chlorella* is a very small amount of food. I personally take 10-12 grams of *Chlorella* a day because I have placed it at the center of my diet, as it should be used. *"Chlorella's main contribution to the body's natural defense system is its beneficial supportive effects on so many of the organs and systems, especially the immune system."* [36]

However, exactly what this CGF substance is still remains a deep mystery. It is an amalgam of RNA, DNA, amino acids, vitamins, minerals and enzymes whose exact properties have not yet been identified. RNA and DNA, both elements of the CGF, facilitate the acceleration of tissue mending. Our cells cannot properly divide and copy themselves without sufficient amounts of RNA and DNA.

"The CGF stimulates repair of tissue damage." [37] This is true even if the tissue has been ulcerated and has resisted traditional healing methods. *Chlorella* is also used effectively as a topical treatment for damaged tissue. Chlorella has the ability to fortify the immune system and heal tissue like no other food known.

Researchers at the Universities of Kanazawa, Japan, and Taipei, Taiwan, conducted a joint study, which was presented at an International Congress at Reims, France in 1985. Tumors subsided in mice when they were given *Chlorella* and *Chlorella* derivatives such as CGF. They concluded that these results came by way of a strengthened immune system. CGF's extraordinary properties help reverse chronic diseases of many kinds.

"Many more studies also demonstrate that Chlorella stimulates the immune system by way of macrophage stimulation." [38]

Research also indicates that *Chlorella* is effective in restoring the body if weakened by persistent hydrocarbon and metallic toxins such as DDT, PCB, mercury, cadmium and lead, while strengthening the immune system response.

CGF improves the immune system and strengthens the body's ability to recover from both exercise and disease. It also helps prevent gastric ulcers and promotes healthy pregnancies. In experiments, mice that were injected with cancer cells showed a high resistance to the cancer when they were fed *Chlorella.* Another experiment showed that CGF improved resistance to abdominal tumors and increased the number of immune cells in the abdominal cavity.

Scientific research indicates that regular use of *Chlorella* prevents heart disease, reduces high blood pressure and serum cholesterol levels. The CGF is also known as *Chlorella* extract.

Chlorella is Alkaline and Helps Balance the Body's pH

It is important that we maintain a balanced body pH, ideally around 6.8 - 7.0, which is about neutral. However, a poor diet of cooked and processed foods forces body pH lower. Nearly all cooked food contributes to the overall acid profile of the body to some degree. Even if it is not raw with its enzymes intact, *Chlorella* is an extremely alkaline food, as is *Spirulina.*

Chlorella & Liver Function

Chlorella has a number of properties, which are helpful to organs and tissue that have been injured by a variety of causes. It has been shown to promote liver health better than any other food. It has been called the *great normalizer*, righting bodily functions that are out of balance.

"Chlorella has also been shown to protect the liver from toxic injury due to ethionine. Ethionine is a drug which induces a fatty liver type of injury much like the liver damage that malnutrition produces. Other studies have shown elevated levels of albumin and decreased levels of globulin while taking Chlorella which is what you would expect to see."[39]

In 1975, Japanese researchers established a link between *Chlorella* intake and lower blood and liver cholesterol. The chlorophyll in *Chlorella* cleanses the liver as well as bowel tissue. Several studies in the US and Japan have revealed the profoundly beneficial effect

Chlorella has on bowel function by helping to carry away toxins, fats and cholesterol from the body, all of which can negatively affect liver health.

"Chlorella's cleansing action on the elimination organs and liver helps keep the blood clean." [40]

It also builds the hemoglobin count in the blood. A clean, smooth-flowing bloodstream rich in oxygen is the foundation of a strong immune system. Along with a healthy digestive and elimination system, strong, rich, toxin-ridding blood will provide great relief for the liver, allowing it to strengthen and cleanse itself

Chlorella, RNA & DNA, and Healing

The high amounts of RNA & DNA in *Chlorella* help repair damaged liver and other bodily tissue at a remarkable rate. Dr. Benjamin Frank theorized that as people age, the resulting loss of energy and physical deterioration was due to the breakdown and decay of nucleic factors such as RNA & DNA, which must be present to keep cells healthy. He fed his patients foods rich in RNA & DNA such as wheat germ, green leafy vegetables, sardines and salmon then published a study illustrating the importance of RNA & DNA in the diet. *Chlorella* contains at least five times more RNA & DNA than any other food, including sardines, which are regarded high in these nucleic substances.

"When our RNA and DNA are in good repair and able to function most efficiently, our bodies get rid of toxins and avoid disease. Cells are able to repair themselves, and the energy level and vitality of the whole body is raised." [41]

"This capacity to promote growth in the young is apparently related to Chlorella's ability to stimulate the healing process in the body and work against many disease states - probably due to its nucleic acid content more than anything else - since the same substances and process that accelerate growth in the young promote repair of damaged tissue in mature animals and humans." [42]

The Most Powerful Food Known

After using sufficient amounts of Chlorella for several years, even long-standing problems such as memory-loss, arthritis and depression will begin to abate. However, *Chlorella* should be used as a *preventative health* measure in order to avoid these problems before they start.

We are constantly exposed to toxins and other pollutants in our environment. Our food is contaminated with both natural and artificial toxins. Heavy metals are present in much of our food because they are found everywhere in nature. However, there are few substances that effectively remove heavy metals and other toxins from the body the way *Chlorella* does. This is why *Chlorella* must be taken everyday! *"Chlorella has great potential in aiding the treatment of cancer, AIDS, Epstein Barr virus and other chronic viral illnesses and is especially helpful in preventing the degenerative diseases associated with the aging process."* [43]

As our soil becomes depleted of its nutrients so will our bodies if we continue to exclusively consume this weakened food. This depletion of nutrients from our food base is beginning to surface in the next generation with alarming statistics such as the rise of obesity and diabetes in children. Considering this, *Spirulina* and *Chlorella* will undoubtedly take on greater significance. *Spirulina* and *Chlorella,* however, are cultured in water, not soil. The proper nutrients can be more easily obtained and utilized in its production because these foods are grown in a controlled environment.

Chlorella Pyrenoidosa
Nutritional Analysis

Moisture (Air oven method)	1.8%
Protein (N x 6.25)	60.8%
Fat (Method with acid hydrolysis)	10.5%
Fiber	3.1%
Ash	6.5%
Non-fibrous carbohydrates	17.3%
*Ratio of pepsin-digestible protein	76.3%
Phosphorus	1.35%
Iron	205 mg/100g
Calcium	345 mg/100g
Potassium	989 mg/100g
Magnesium	331 mg/100g

*Test condition:0.2%pepsin(activity 1:10,000), incubation with shaking for 16 hr at 45 C

T-BHC.. none
DDT.. detected(MLD
*0.01 ppm)
Aerobic plate count.. (MLD 0.1
Coagulase positive Staphylococci.. mg/100g)
Coliform Bacteria .... none
detected(MLD
0.02 ppm)
(MLD 0.1
mg/100g)
negative/2.22g
negative/0.01g

*MLD: Minimum limit of determination

Carotene	32.1 mg/100g
Thiamin (equivalent to Thiamin	1.56 mg/100g
Hydrochloride)	4.49 mg/100g

Riboflavin	1.94 mg/100g
Vitamin B6	38 mg/100g
Total ascorbic acid	5.9 mg/100g
Tocopherol	5.7 mg/100g
A-Tocopherol	0.2 mg/100g
B-Tocopherol	none detected
T-Tocopherol	(MLD 0.1
8-Tocopherol	mg/100g)
	none detected
Folic acid	(MLD 0.1
Niacin	mg/100g)
Total chlorophyll	1.0 mg/100g
*2 Xanthophyll	26.5 mg/100g
	2.17%
	302 mg/100g

*1 MLD: Minimum limit of determination
*2 The xanthophyll contents were calculated from =1,800 (at 453nm, chloroform) as standard

Amino acids

Arginine	3.49%
Lysine	3.29%
Histidine	1.14%
Phenylalanine	2.77%
Tyrosine	2.03%
Leucine	4.81%
Isoleucine	2.21%
Methionine*	1.41%
Valine	3.33%
Alanine	4.58%
Glycine	3.23%
Proline	2.60%
Glutamic acid	6.02%
Serine	2.29%
Threonine	2.70%
Aspartic acid	5.06%
Tryptophan	1.11%
*Cystine	0.69%

Total pheophorbides (KANSHOKU No.99).....................	12 %
Original pheophorbide..	7 %
Chlorophyllase activity..	5 %

*By Hydrochloric acid hydrolysis after performic acid oxidation.

Chapter 6

Spirulina

(Spirulina Pacifica)

Nature's Perfect Energy Food

"A lie can travel halfway around the world while the truth is putting on its shoes."

~ Mark Twain

Occasionally, I will hear someone refer to algae as pond scum. I even hear it from nutritionists from time to time and it is a scurrilous lie.

Spirulina Magnified 650X

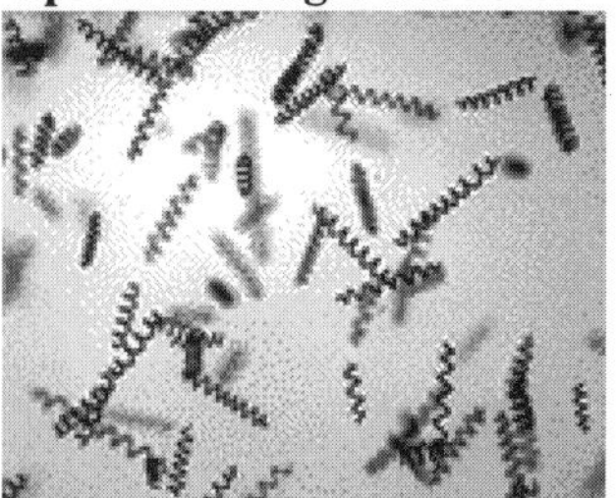

Spirulina Pacifica is a blue green micro-algae and one of the two most powerful whole foods on Earth. Like *Chlorella,* it is extremely nutritious and can be eaten by anyone at any age. *Spirulina Pacifica* is a microscopic freshwater plant grown only in Hawaii, an aquatic micro-vegetable/ organism composed of transparent bubble-thin cells stacked end-to-end, forming a helical spiral filament. *Spirulina's* exterior cell wall is comprised of complex organic sugars that are easily digested, thus the cell wall does not need to be broken open as it does with *Chlorella*. *Spirulina* is about 60% protein containing 18 amino acids and is a vastly superior protein source to any other food, including meat, which has only 11 amino acids. *Spirulina* contains more beta-carotene and GLA (gamma linolenic acid) than any other whole food. It contains 92 trace minerals and other elements such as vitamins, chlorophyll, glyolipids, phycocyanin, carotenoids and sulfolipids. It is also high in superoxide dismutase (SOD), RNA and DNA, which have only recently been identified as essential nutrients. While *Spirulina* does not contain all the nutrients the body needs, one could easily live on nothing else and expect to be completely healthy. It is less than four calories per gram and has almost no cholesterol.

Spirulina Pacifica is a superior strain of *Spirulina* compared to other strains such as *Spirulina Plantensis.* It contains three times the beta carotene, twice the SOD, ten times the calcium and four times the iron than other *Spirulina* strains. It is cultivated using advanced techniques of strain selection, which further refines the algae with each generation.

Proteins are fundamental components of all living cells and include various materials and substances such as enzymes, antibodies and hormones that are vital for the proper functioning of all organisms. They are essential nutrients in our diet for growth and tissue repair and are found in foods such as meat, fish, eggs, dairy products, legumes and algae. *Spirulina's* broad array of amino acids (protein) provides the body with an abundance of energy because amino acids are the building blocks of our cells. When our cells receive the nutrients they require, they can properly perform their myriad functions throughout the body and we naturally feel more energetic.

Spirulina produces all its nutrients by harvesting sunlight. It gathers and transforms sunlight into green and blue pigments that make it a blue green algae. The blue is an amino acid group found only in *Spirulina* called phycocyanin, which accounts for its high concentration of vegetarian protein. The green in *Spirulina* is chlorophyll, one of the best natural detoxifiers known.

Spirulina is an extremely high energy food. It contains all the B vitamins, which are themselves synonymous with high energy. Energy derived from whole foods such as *Spirulina* and *Chlorella* is natural and will never leave you flat after their nutrients have been consumed by the body. Scientific studies worldwide have demonstrated the incredible cancer prevention properties of *Spirulina,* such as its high levels of beta carotene.

Water, nitrogen, phosphorus, carbon dioxide and sunlight are all that is needed to produce *Spirulina*, one of the most nutritionally packed foods in the world, an absolutely astounding array of enzymes and other nutrients.

Having a copper deficiency, for instance, is responsible in part for people's hair turning gray because it leads to a deficiency in the enzyme reaction that produces hair pigment. However, taking a supplement with copper in it will not provide sufficient copper to the body to arrest the decline of this enzymatic process. *Spirulina* contains a lot of copper and all its minerals are bio-chelated, meaning they are naturally wrapped in amino acids so they will be readily absorbed by the body.

And because they are bio-chelated, they will never build up in the body and become toxic.

Spirulina is often used in smoothie drinks and added to nutrition bars in order to fortify it with nutrients. It has a seaweed-like taste that many people find unpleasant, which is why it is best taken in 100% pure tabletted form.

Algae was the first food on the planet billions of years ago. It turned our carbon-dioxide atmosphere in to an oxygen breathing atmosphere, which laid the foundation for the myriad insects, animals and mammals that would one day inhabit the planet. Life evolved out of this environment and from algae itself, which is why certain species of algae are such perfect foods.

There are over 32,000 species of algae on Earth. Some contain deadly poisons and toxins, others are incredible foods packed with nutrients found nowhere else in nature. And while there are many other algae that are suitable as a food source, only *Spirulina* and *Chlorella* have the power that few whole foods, including other algae, come close to.

Spirulina has a Long History and Bright Future

Spirulina has been eaten by many cultures throughout history. The Aztecs and Mayas used *Spirulina* as a central part of their diet. The Kanembu people, who live along the shores of Lake Chad, still use it today. NASA considers *Spirulina* an ideal food and plans to grow and use it on long-term space flights. It will be one of the first foods grown on the Space Station. *Spirulina* is one of the most efficient, oxygen-generating foods in existence. It is extremely easy to grow and takes less room per cubic centimeter than any other crop known, yielding an enormous amount of nutrition.

Spirulina and *Chlorella* are ideal foods to feed a starving world. They have been used in Third World Countries to relieve hunger with great effectiveness because they are inexpensive, nutritionally compact and not given to quick spoilage.

You will never find a better nutritional buy anywhere on the market than you will with both *Spirulina* and *Chlorella*. *Ounce for ounce, your dollar goes farther toward providing the body with proper nutrition than any other foods available.* There are a lot of different *Spirulina* brands on the market. A rule of thumb is to only buy

Spirulina Pacifica that is Certified Organic, ISO 9200 (international standards) and Certified Kosher.

Spirulina is Pure Food

Spirulina has a 95% digestibility rate compared with only 3-7% for most cooked foods, and 55%-75% for most raw foods. It is higher than any other food, including *Chlorella,* which is 80% digestible. However, *Chlorella* is comprised of 20% fiber. *Spirulina* does not have nearly the amount of fiber in it that *Chlorella* has. *Spirulina* is a whole food unlike vitamins and other supplements. Nothing has been added to *Spirulina* or extracted from another source to produce it. Most multiple vitamins sold on the market are comprised of laboratory synthesized chemical compounds and are not derived from natural sources. Virtually all vitamins are amalgams of extracts and concentrates, some of which can accumulate in the body and become toxic, especially if they are fat soluble. This is particularly true if they have been synthesized. Organic whole foods are *never* toxic.

The other problem with the vitamin approach to nutrition is that vitamin companies foolishly attempt to duplicate, reinvent or improve on nature, which of course can never be done. One reason is that natural whole foods contain an abundance of enzymes, something that cannot be artificially reproduced. Given the amount of nutrition they provide, vitamin supplements are also considerably more expensive.

Spirulina is a balanced natural whole food. It contains over 100 synergistic nutrients and is nature's richest and most complete source of total organic nutrition. *Spirulina* is a completely natural, and therefore superior, approach to nutrition.

Spirulina Shown Helpful for Arthritis

Spirulina is a rich source of Gamma Linolenic Acid (GLA), which is the miracle ingredient in *Spirulina.* GLA is an essential fatty acid that has been shown quite helpful in the relief of arthritis.

GLA helps lower high blood pressure and blood cholesterol. It is used in treating degenerative diseases, premenstrual syndrome, eczema and other skin conditions. Mother's milk and *Spirulina* are the only natural whole foods where GLA is found.

Spirulina Is Nature's Richest Whole Food Source of Organic Iron

The iron in *Spirulina* is completely nontoxic, meaning that it will not build up in the body and become poisonous the way commercial or synthetic iron supplements can. Gram per gram, it is 58 times richer in organic iron than raw spinach and 28 times richer than raw beef liver. Three grams of *Spirulina* contains the equivalent amount of iron as 80 grams of liver or two cups of raw spinach. Iron is used in cell production and in various other places in the body. There is an iron molecule at the center of every human blood cell, thus the importance of iron in human health cannot be minimized.

Iron deficiency amongst women is quite common, mainly because of the loss of iron during menstruation. Child bearing women and vegetarians are particularly at risk of having low iron.

The fact that *Spirulina's* iron is biochelated, naturally wrapped in amino acids, means that it more easily assimilates into the body. The iron found in vitamin supplements is not nearly as bio-available to the body as the iron found in *Spirulina*. In fact, only about 10% of the iron found in supplements is absorbed and used by the body. The rest either passes or accumulates in unwanted places throughout the body, especially in the organs.

Spirulina contains Phycocyanin and Glycolipids

Phycocyanin, the natural blue pigment in *Spirulina*, is not found in any other food. Phycocyanin has been used in cancer treatments and helps stimulate the immune system. It is used in the treatment of renal failure, even that resulting from the side-effects of drug therapies. Glycolipids have been extracted from *Spirulina* and used in the treatment of AIDS. These nutrients have just recently begun to be studied and found to be extremely useful to human health.

Powerful Nutraceutical

A nutraceutical is a food that provides the body with the proper nutrients so the body can heal itself, which it certainly can do if provided with the right materials, or nutrients, to do the job. There are many foods that have healing and *preventative health* qualities, but none possess such a powerful, wide-ranging and diverse group of nutrients as *Spirulina* and *Chlorella*. *Spirulina* contains every natural known antioxidant including zinc, manganese, selenium and copper, the amino acid methionine, vitamins E, A, C, B-1, B-2, B-6, B-12 and beta-carotene.

Nature's Richest Source of Vitamin B-12

Spirulina has more vitamin B-12 than any other whole food source. It is 4-6 times richer than raw beef liver, it's nearest rival. Vitamin B-12 is famous for providing the human body with high energy and is used in the treatment of anemia. Vitamin B-12 is found in meat. It is difficult for vegetarians to get sufficient doses of Vitamin B-12 from other foods. *Spirulina* contains an abundance of B-12 as well as the entire vitamin B complex. It is important when taking one B vitamin that all of them be taken with it because they are dependent upon one another to function to their fullest capacity.

Contains Natural Digestive and Other Enzymes

Over two thousand different enzymes have been identified in *Spirulina*. Enzymes are a critical component of good health and the shear variety that are in *Spirulina* makes it one of the best enzymes sources available. Like *Chlorella, Spirulina* has been scientifically proven to increase the reproduction of lactobacilli, the friendly bacteria that helps digest our food.

Contains SOD (Super Oxide Dismutase)

SOD is one of most powerful antioxidants known, which assists the cell in renewing itself. It is an enzyme our body must have in order to function properly. This essential enzyme is crucial to the body's ability to assimilate amino acids (protein). Without the presence of SOD in the body, we are unable to create the hundreds of thousands of long, complex chains of amino acids that form proteins. SOD is found in very few foods in nature, yet is highly concentrated in *Spirulina*.

Richest Whole Food Source Of Vitamin E and Beta Carotene (Pro Vitamin A)

Spirulina contains more beta carotene than any other whole food. It produces beta carotene and other carotenoids to protect itself from the sun. The more intense the sunlight, the more beta carotene is produced. Beta carotene determines how our cells communicate with one another. *"Beta carotene opens the membrane communication channels of cancerous and pre-cancerous cells, allowing the body to signal the cancerous cells to stop dividing. Therefore, foods rich in beta carotene may not only be able to prevent but also reverse cancers."*[44]

Anyone with cancer or having a high risk of getting cancer should consider taking large doses of beta-carotene. Research has demonstrated that beta-carotene can lower cholesterol, treat wounds and reduce the size of tumors. Natural beta-carotene is far superior to synthetic, both chemically and physically. It is absorbed easier than synthetics and it will not build up in the body and become toxic. Instead, the body efficiently stores it for future use. The body will not store synthetic beta-carotene. These man-made versions often contain preservatives and other chemical residues.

There are no toxic side effects of any kind when consuming Spirulina. Unlike the preformed synthetic vitamin A and fish liver oil extracts, beta-carotene is completely nontoxic, even in mega doses. Beta carotene is a strong antioxidant and cancer fighter. It is only one of over 600 different carotenoids. Carotenoids are used throughout the body including the spleen, pancreas, skin, reproductive system, adrenal glands and retina.

Spirulina has three times the vitamin E than that of raw wheat germ and its biological activity is 49% greater than synthetic vitamin E. It has 25 times the Beta Carotene than that of raw carrots.

Powerful Natural Detoxifier

Spirulina has a cleansing effect that works first on the digestive system, then the blood and finally the entire body after several months of consistent use. It has several organic chemical substances that promote detoxification, including chlorophyll. The shear size of this micro-algae has a detoxifying effect on our cells.

Complete Protein

Spirulina has all the eight essential amino acids as well as ten others, thus it is considered a complete protein, unlike meat. Like *Chlorella,* it is 60% protein and contains 18 out of the 22 known amino acids. This is why *Spirulina* is such an incredibly valuable food source to vegetarians.

It is very important that the human body has all of the amino acids available to form the hundreds of thousands of complex proteins that it requires. If some of the amino acids are not present, the result is incomplete protein formation. These truncated proteins do not function as effectively or efficiently as they would if all the amino acids were present. Entire pieces of these proteins will be missing without all the amino acids present and their service to the body greatly diminished. Our body's life force, the ongoing dynamic enzymatic processes, depend directly upon the presence and proper formation of complex proteins. Life ceases without the presence of amino acids.

Most animal protein contains large amounts of fat, which *Spirulina* does not. Fat can impede the formation of proteins from amino acids.

Helps Balance your Body's pH

Spirulina, like *Chlorella*, is one of the most alkaline foods that can be eaten. This is true despite the fact that both are 60% amino acids, which are of course acidic by nature.

All green foods such as kale, spinach, greens, asparagus and broccoli are alkaline. Keeping the body's pH balanced is achieved much easier with detoxifying green foods such as *Spirulina*.

Weight Loss and Sports Training

Spirulina is a rich, natural source of phenylalanine-slimmers. It effectively suppresses the appetite. Its whole food nutrition facilitates low-calorie dieting without the energy draining and health destroying nutritional deficiencies that are the downfall of most weight-loss programs. *Spirulina* satisfies hunger because it fulfills the body's basic nutritional and biochemical needs. Most multiple vitamin/mineral supplements today are laboratory-synthesized chemical compounds that cannot provide the basic nutritional building blocks that raw foods such as *Spirulina* and *Chlorella* do.

According to internationally acclaimed author and nutritionist Dr. Paavo Airola: "*It is wisest and safest to take vitamins and minerals in the form of food supplements where they occur in their natural form and strength, and in combination with all of the other nutritive factors such as enzymes and trace elements, for optimum assimilation and biological activity."*

Foods that are eaten in their raw state with their enzymes intact are assimilated into the body with many times the usefulness and efficiency of foods that have been cooked, freeze dried, pasteurized or otherwise processed.

Fitness enthusiasts, body-builders, professional coaches and competitive athletes' report increased energy, enhanced endurance, recovery and overall improved performance with *Spirulina* and *Chlorella.* I can testify to this myself.

Hundreds of Olympic and world champion athletes use *Spirulina* both during training and competition. Olympian Lee Evans, double gold medallist and holder of four world records in track and field, says: "*Spirulina improved my training, resulting in faster times. It increased my stamina and endurance."* Now as a coach, Lee demands all his athletes use *Spirulina*.

Spirulina Production: Cultured vs. Wild

Algae grows everywhere in the world. It is impossible to get rid of, thank goodness, because if algae ever disappeared, so would all life on Earth. Algae, not the rain forest, generate most of the oxygen in the Earth's atmosphere as is often misreported. Algae is at the very bottom of the food chain because it was the first food to appear on the planet 2.5 billion years ago. The more ancient the food the more nutritionally compact and broader array of nutrients are likely contained in it. We essentially evolved as a species over billions of years out of algae, which is why these foods are more nutritious for us than any others.

One of the great advantages of cultivated crops over wild crops is that cultivated strains are grown in a way that refines, strengthens and develops the strain to its greatest nutritional benefit. Rice, for instance, is wild grass that has been cultivated over thousands of years and become so refined and successful that today's rice strains have the ability to feed hungry nations with their abundance.

Algae such AFA that are harvested from an uncontrolled lake environment do not have anything close to the nutritional potential compared to a strain of cultivated *Spirulina Pacifica* that has been refined over thousands of generations in a controlled environment.

Hawaii has the best growing environment for *Spirulina* in the world. Aquaculturists select from millions of *Spirulina* cells in order to develop superior strains of microalgae that are higher in nutrients such as beta carotene, iron, amino acids, calcium and numerous others.

Cultivated algae is farmed in huge ponds from live culture, which essentially is the seed from which the algae crop is grown. The algae is covered with a layer of natural calcium carbonate. Sea water is used to grow *Spirulina Pacifica* so all the minerals from the sea are found in Hawaiian *Spirulina*. Giant paddle wheels gently turn the algae in order to ensure optimum light exposure for each cell. This also helps release tremendous amounts of oxygen, which is good for the environment.

Cultivated algae grows very rapidly, several times that of wild algae. *Spirulina* farming operations typically produce over 200,000 pounds (91,000 kg) of *Spirulina* per year on only fifteen acres of land. Since *Spirulina* is 60% protein, that calculates to a staggering 120,000 pounds (54,500 kg) of protein per year or 8,000 pounds per acre. This far exceeds the yield of other high protein crops such as triticale grain, kamu and even soybeans. The amount of protein derived from cattle per acre is negligible compared with that of either *Spirulina* or *Chlorella*.

Algae is also a much cleaner crop to produce since there is no manure or fertilizer used to grow the algae. Thus there is no possibility of contamination from commercial manure or chemical fertilizers and of course there is no run off pollution from them. Hawaiian *Spirulina* is always grown herbicide and pesticide free! Don't settle for anything less than Certified Organic *Spirulina*.

Harvesting, Drying and Tableting *Spirulina*

The only thing easier than cultivating *Spirulina* is harvesting it. In fact, the hardest thing about producing *Spirulina* is refining, strengthening and purifying the strain. That is where the real expertise comes into play when growing algae.

Spirulina is harvested in giant stainless steel screens because it's filamentous, meaning that is grows in long twisting strands. This method of harvesting *Spirulina* allows the delicate cells and its nutrients to remain intact. It is then washed with fresh water several times. Only half of the cultivation ponds are harvested, the other half left behind as seed for the next generation.

Once harvested, *Spirulina* must then be dried. There are three methods of drying currently used. Freeze drying, spray drying and Ocean-Chill Drying (US Patent #5,276,977). Freeze drying is convenient and inexpensive, but it destroys the most important part of the food, the enzymes. Freeze drying exposes the algae to large amounts of oxygen, which also destroys the enzymes and other vital nutrients. The algae is also exposed to very high temperatures at the end of the freeze drying process. Although it was used frequently decades ago as a drying process, freeze drying is rarely used today. AFA lake harvested algae uses freeze drying because it destroys the huge amounts of bacteria that are harvested with the algae. These high levels of bacteria do not exist in controlled environment algae cultivation ponds such as those used to produce *Spirulina Pacifica*.

Spray drying has been used in *Spirulina* production for many years because it is quick and effective, drying the algae in seconds. However, because it also uses high temperatures, there is a significant danger of destroying the delicate and crucial enzymes of the algae. Because of this danger, Ocean-Chill Drying was developed utilizing extremely cold sea water from a depth of 2000 feet which removes the moisture and chills the air in the dryer. This dehumidifying effect removes oxygen from the dryer, which retains nutrients such as beta carotene and phycocyanin, but most importantly it allows the enzymes to remain fully intact. Ocean-Chill Drying is by far the greatest advance in *Spirulina* production in decades.

Tabletting the algae is the final process and the last chance for nutrient and enzyme damage, thus steps must be taken to insure there is no degradation in the nutritional content of the algae. The most cost effective and quickest way is to add binders or excipients to the algae powder, however this exposes the algae to oxidation, which destroys the nutrients. Another method used is called granulation, which moistens the algae then heats it in trays for hours, which also destroys enzymes and other nutrients.

Although it is the most costly and time consuming, the best method for tabletting *Spirulina* or *Chlorella* is to run the tablet presses at very low heat. This provides for a tabletted algae that has not had its enzymes or nutritional profile damaged in any way.

Chlorella is harvested using a different method known as centrifugation, which is much more costly. It also must have its cell wall broken open, which *Spirulina* does not. Thus *Chlorella* tends to be slightly more expensive than *Spirulina*.

Between the two of them, a broader array of nutrients for the human body cannot be found anywhere.

Hawaiian Spirulina Pacifica

Nutritional Analysis

GENERAL COMPOSITION	
Protein	60%
Carbohydrates	19%
Lipids	6%
Minerals	8%
Moisture	7%

VITAMINS	
Beta-carotene	10 mg
Vitamin A (100% as Beta-Carotene)	15,030 IU
Vitamin B1 (Thiamin)	102 mcg
Vitamin B2 (Riboflavin)	99 mcg
Vitamin B3 (Niacin)	621 mcg
Vitamin B6	13.2 mcg
Vitamin B12	6.6 mcg
Inositol	2.04 mg
Biotin	0.969 mg
Folic Acid	0.9 mcg
Pantothenic Acid	12 mcg

FATTY ACIDS	
Omega 6 Family	
Gamma Linolenic (GLA)	30 mg
Essential Linolenic	33 mg
Dihomogamma Linolenic	1.59 mg
Omega 3 Family	
Alpha Linolenic	0.0435 mg
Docosahexaenoic (DHA)	0.0435 mg
Monoenoic Family	
Palmitoleic	5.94 mg

Oleic	0.51 mg
Erucic	0.072 mg

MINERALS	
Calcium	12 mg
Magnesium	14.4 mg
Iron	3.18 mg
Phosphorous	31.2 mg
Potassium	45.6 mg
Sodium	21.9 mg
Manganese	78 mcg
Zinc	36 mcg
Boron	30 mcg
Copper	3 mcg
Molybdenum	3 mcg

PHYTONUTRIENTS	
Beta-carotene 9-*cis*	1.60 mg
Beta-carotene 13-*cis*	0.51 mg
Beta-carotene 15-*cis*	0.12 mg
Beta-carotene all-*trans*	7.80 mg
Zeaxanthin	0.95 mg
Chlorophyll	23.70 mg
Total carotenoids*	14 mg
Phycocyanin	333 mg
Superoxide Dismutase**	2640 units
*Includes alpha carotene, beta cryptoxanthin & others. **Reported as units Ferric S.O.D.	

Chapter 7
Biomagnets and their Applied Therapies

"Nothing astonishes men so much as common sense and plain dealing."

~ Ralph Waldo Emerson

Until now, I have only discussed nutrition and water in this book, what we can and should put in our body to achieve Great Health. However, I have included this discussion on the use of biomagnets because of their strong benefit to our health. Biomagnets can and should be used by everyone, even animals. Magnetic therapy will one day become as common as any other form of medical treatment. Biomagnets are extremely effective in helping the body heal, and maintain a healthy profile.

Negative pole magnetic fields penetrate the surface of the body and affect the nervous system, cells and organs in a beneficial way. Like *Ionized Water*, if employed properly the use of magnetic field therapy has no known negative or harmful side effects. Magnetic therapy has been used effectively to combat arthritis and rheumatoid diseases, bone fractures, insomnia, headaches and migraines, cancer, tumors, circulatory disease and related problems, knotted muscles, carpal tunnel syndrome (repetitive motion syndrome), infections and pain of almost any other kind.

"The healing potential of magnets is possible because the body's nervous system is governed, in part, by varying patterns of ionic currents and electromagnetic fields." [46]

The *negative North Pole* (green side) has an allaying effect that restores proper metabolic balance to the body or area of the body where it is applied. The *positive South Pole* (red side) disrupts metabolic balance and function, depletes oxygen in the cells, produces acid and promotes the growth of dormant microorganisms in the body.

Magnetic fields have tremendous positive effects on the human body. Sleeping in a bed with the head pointed north will provide you with a better night's sleep than if its pointed in a different direction, especially east or west. It may sound like an old wife's tale, but it works because the magnetic field of the earth will flow around the body and not hit it from the side, which is a very subtle difference that can have profound repercussions on overall sleep patterns.

The strength of a magnet is measured in units of *gauss*. The higher the *gauss* level, the stronger the magnet. Good biomagnets will have a *gauss* level of 2,000-3,400, meaning it is a magnet strong enough to be therapeutic. When using magnets as therapeutic tools, the negative north (green) pole should *always* be placed toward the skin. Magnetic strength quickly diminishes with distance so they should be placed directly against the skin.

Magnets have been used therapeutically for thousands of years and can be traced back to Chinese medicine. Paraclesus, the Father of Medicine, regularly prescribed magnetic therapy for all sorts of pain and was ridiculed by his colleagues for doing so; however, he was the first medical professional to explain magnetic therapy in relation to body chemistry, thus removing the idea that magnets were alchemy and therefore unsubstantiated.

The medical establishment has roundly dismissed magnetic therapy. However, medical institutions are conducting research on biomagnets, some with FDA approved electromagnetic therapies.

"The biochemical mechanism present in the human body can be viewed as a matrix of billions of cells that run on minute electrical currents. When the human battery is charged, the body's electrical system is working properly. Biomagnetism increases the body's natural energy systems. When the body's vitality is elevated, rapid healing of many illnesses, diseases and painful physical conditions occurs naturally."[47]

TMS, *Transcrannial Magnetic Stimulation,* has been used successfully to fight depression and other related mental diseases and is currently being studied at several major medical hospitals around the country.

Drinking negatively charged water is also good for one's health. Placing the negative North Pole of a strong magnet against a water glass for 10-15 minutes will magnetize the water for 15-20 hours. This causes the ions in the water to become negatively charged, meaning they are all spinning in the same direction. The reason this water is beneficial to us when we drink it is because the body is more able to metabolize the oxygen and hydrogen atoms that are in the water when it is South Pole magnetized. This is because water that has been magnetized provides the same charge to all the electrons, which separates the atoms thus making the oxygen and hydrogen more bioavailable.

In his book, Young Again, John Thomas speaks of the importance of maintaining a predominance of negatively spinning ions in the body because this is how it optimally functions in a negative ion environment. He correctly warns us against consuming *canola* or *rapeseed oil* because it is a substance that has a positive ion spin, which runs counter to the natural state of the body.

We drink *Ionized Water* for the negative ions and it is for this same reason that *Negative Ion Generators* are beneficial for air purification and mood elevation. They flood the room with negative ions, thus creating an environment that is more conducive to human health. Negative ions are found in great abundance in the mountains, especially near waterfalls. It was never the *mountain air* that made people feel better when they pilgrimaged to the mountains, seeking to alleviate health problems, but what actually was *in the air, Negative Ions*.

PART THREE
Chapter 8
Youth, Maturation and Reversing the Aging Process

"Youth is a wonderful thing. What a crime it is to waste it on children."

~ GB Shaw.

When we talk about *Reversing the Aging Process,* we can only be referring to renewal of the body's cells. The most efficient and natural way to achieve this is to drink *Ionized Water* and provide the body with the exact nutrients and enzymes it needs.

There are several reverse aging theories and treatments currently being proposed and experimented with. Some approaches have met with limited success.

Often overlooked, however, is the importance of detoxification. Toxins are everywhere in our environment. Some toxins are artificial, others naturally occurring. Heavy metals, for instance, are naturally found throughout the food chain. They accumulate in wild animals the same way they do in humans, although usually to a much lesser extent. When humans suffer from heavy metal poisoning, it is usually caused by something unnatural such as mercury from teeth fillings, lead pipes, or aluminum from cans, antiperspirants or antacids.

Simply put, toxins are elements that do not belong in the human body. As we age, these foreign substances accumulate in our brain tissue, body tissue and organs. Many toxins, for instance, are found in the medicine that we take, both over the counter and prescription. We need to spend each day of our lives detoxifying ourselves, cleansing the body of the elements that are alien to it. Detoxification needs to be an ongoing process, something that ideally becomes a part of our daily lives. Here are a few excellent methods of detoxification that can be used.

Ionized Water

Detoxification essentially begins with water and there is none better to detoxify with than *Ionized Water*. We should purge ourselves daily by eating well in the morning then waiting an hour or so before drinking a lot of water to purge or clean ourselves out. Water cleanses the lining of the digestive tract so nutrients can be better absorbed. Keeping this clean will result in better overall health by helping to prevent hemorrhoids, intestinal blockages and even cancer.

Ionized Water's superior hydration properties push toxins out of bodily tissue more effectively than any other substance. Although the detoxifying effects of *Ionized Water* will be felt immediately, it will take months, even years of drinking *Ionized Water* to completely cleanse the body with it.

Chlorella & Spirulina

These are two of the most powerful detoxifiers known. The shear size of micro-algae lend themselves to detoxification because they are able to penetrate and attack disease and toxins in ways other foods and nutrients cannot. *Besides this, both Spirulina* and *Chlorella* contain many chemical substances and enzymes, which detoxify the body, including chlorophyll. *Chlorella's* outer cell wall is comprised of a unique fiber that has the ability to bind with and pull heavy metals and other synthetic toxins out of the body.

Raw Fruits and Vegetables & Herbs

Toxins are more easily deposited in the body by cooked food rather than raw foods that have their enzymes intact. While it is true that you will get detoxification from the chemical substances that many foods contain even after they have been cooked, foods that are consumed raw have far more powerful detoxification potential than foods that are cooked. Many herbs also have strong detoxification properties and should be consumed raw whenever possible.

Far Infra Red Saunas & Clothing

Sweating is one of the best ways to detoxify the skin and its pores. Preferably, one should work up a good sweat everyday by vigorously exercising. Far Infrared light, FIR, is another excellent method of skin detoxification because it heats the skin up, but not the surrounding air. FIR saunas allow the body to sweat profusely without the danger of overheating it or the skin. FIR clothing is also available, which also makes the skin sweat without actually heating the air around it.

Fasting

An excellent way to detoxify is to stop eating and drink only water, preferably *Ionized Water*, anywhere from several hours to several weeks depending on your goals and tenacity. Fasting with distilled, purified or reverse osmosis can be quite dangerous since in the absence of any buffers, this water quickly depletes the body of its minerals and other vital elements. Fasting with distilled water has been known to turn a person's hair gray within weeks because of the severe and sudden loss of copper, which controls hair pigment. This is only an indication of what it is doing to the rest of the body. When fasting, always use caution and drink only spring, mineral or *Ionized Water* that is pH balanced.

Common Sense Ways to Fight Cancer

Let food be your medicine and medicine your food. -- Hippocrates

Theories abound about the source of cancer, how it starts, how it spreads and what can be done to stop it. Some theorize cancer stems from a bacteria or viral infection. Others suggest that it is strictly genetic, inherited from generations past. Others insist that toxins, chemicals, other forms of pollution, and even the human cell reverting back to an embryonic state cause cancer.

However cancer does actually begin, one fact is indisputable: *Cancer, like any other disease, requires an acidic environment to thrive in.* What creates an acid environment in our bodies is a diet of cooked, pasteurized, processed foods and other highly acid activities such as smoking, drinking liquor and the most acid activity of all, consuming soft drinks.

There are natural, commonsense activities someone with cancer can engage in to help fight the disease. Keep in mind, however, that they work best as *preventative health* measures.

Consume *Ionized Water*

There are several good reasons to drink *Ionized Water* to help fight cancer. First, it is very alkaline and anything that can be done to keep the body more alkaline will help fight the cancer. Cancer thrives in an acid environment so it creates an ever more acid environment for itself to live in. Cancer patients near death often smell bad because their body has created ammonia (which is alkaline) as a natural chemical response to the onslaught of acid that is attacking it.

Second, *Ionized Water* provides the body with a great deal of oxygen. Higher blood oxygen levels from drinking *Ionized Water* are common and can even be expected. *Ionized Water* is akin to drinking liquid oxygen and *oxygen kills cancer cells.* Cancer patients are often tired because the cancer has depleted their oxygen. By drinking *Ionized Water*, the body is being provided with an abundance of oxygen that will kill the cancer cells, give the patient more energy and a greater overall potential to fight the disease.

The negative ORP (mV) of *Ionized Water* will also create a less conducive environment in the body for cancer to thrive in. Cancer, like any other disease, has a natural tendency to thrive best in a high ORP environment.

The detoxification effects of *Ionized Water* will also help flush the cancer cells from the body. Once acclimated to it, one can never drink too much *Ionized Water*. One to two gallons or more per day is an appropriate amount of *Ionized Water* for someone with cancer to consume. Remember, however, to never drink water around mealtime.

Take large doses of *Chlorella* and *Spirulina*

Chlorella has many anti-cancer properties. It causes the body to produce *interferon*, one of the body's strongest natural defense mechanisms used to prevent and fight cancer. *Chlorella* is also very alkaline. The wide array of amino acids found in *Chlorella* form proteins the body needs. However, the protein found in *Chlorella* is not dangerous to cancer patients who are advised by physicians not to consume too much protein such as meat.

While *Spirulina does* not have the powerful cancer-fighting agents that *Chlorella* has, it certainly should not be overlooked. *Spirulina* is also very alkaline and considered a nutraceutical. Like *Chlorella*, it has thousands of different enzymes that have been identified in it. It has more beta-carotene than any other food, which is known for having strong anti-cancer properties.

A dosage of 20-25 grams of *Chlorella* and 15-20 grams of *Spirulina* is recommended for someone with a disease as serious as cancer.

Eat Raw Fruits and Vegetables

Incorporate these foods into your diet

Raw foods have many advantages over cooked foods. The less cooked food a cancer patient eats, the better. Raw foods are alkaline, bio-available, detoxifying and carry with them a negative charge (ORP). Each of the following foods contains a chemical substance or enzyme, which has substantial anti-cancer properties:

Anticancer Chemical Substance or Enzyme	Found in which Foods
Carotenoids	Carrots, Green Leafy Vegetables, Sweet Potatoes
Allylic Sulfides	Garlic, Onions, Chives, Leaks
Ellagic Acid	Grapes, Strawberries, Raspberries, Walnuts
Catechins	Berries
Coumarins	Carrots, Parsley, Citrus Fruits
Isothiocyanates	Mustard, Horseradish, Radishes, other Cruciferous Vegetables
Indoles	Cabbage, Broccoli, Cauliflower, Kale, Brussels Sprouts
Lignans	Soybeans, Flaxseed
Protease Inhibitors	Soybeans, Legumes, Nuts, Grains, Seeds
Limoinoids	Citrus Fruit
Sulforaphane	Broccoli, Broccoli Sprouts, Green Onions, Kale, Red Cabbage, Brussels Sprouts, Ginger, Cauliflower, Red-leaf Lettuce

Stop Eating Junk and Avoid Certain Other Foods

Cancer patients should avoid eating alfalfa sprouts because they contain an enzyme that encourages cancer. Dairy products should be avoided completely, as should meat, wheat products and eggs. Soft drinks are *definitely* off the list and should be considered *forever* removed, even if the disease subsides. Anything containing refined flour or sugar should be avoided, which includes 85% of all processed foods. All these things, including cooked foods, will encourage an overall acidic profile in the body, causing the cancer to flourish. Poor diet is often what helps put cancer patients in their situation to begin with. A person must desire to conquer a disease strongly enough to change bad habits. After all, without quality of health, life is substantially diminished. None of the activities suggested above should in any way be considered a cure for cancer, but simply ways to strengthen the body so it can fight the disease that has invaded it. Proper exercise and a positive mental attitude are also essential in fighting disease. One should always immediately seek the advice of medical professionals when confronted with any disease.

Chapter 9

The Three Pillars of *Great Health*

"When you go through hardships and decide not to surrender, that is strength."

~ Arnold Schwarzenegger

The Three Pillars of Great Health are adequate **Water** and proper **Nutrition**, regular **Exercise** and maintaining a **Positive Mental & Spiritual Attitude**. We have talked about the first pillar of health, *Water and Nutrition*, at length in this book. However, the other two pillars are every bit as important because they complete the health picture, and without them Great Health is not obtainable.

Regular Exercise

The human body needs to be exercised everyday. Ideally, the exercise should be moderate to vigorous and last at least 30 minutes. One of the primary benefits of regular exercise is that it cleanses the body, removes toxins and *builds the immune system in ways that nutrients cannot fortify it.* People who exercise regularly are sick much less often than people who do not.

Exercise gets the heart and lungs pumping and the blood circulating. The benefits of all our bodily systems operating vigorously is detoxification, both from sweating and increased circulation of the blood through organs that remove toxins. Exercise helps keep our organs vital and youthful, which of course promotes overall health by keeping the body in balance.

One important aspect of Great Health related to exercise is that of *stretching*. Although its importance is neglected, proper stretching promotes circulation, breathing and a host of other health benefits, including mood elevation. A 75-year old world champion martial arts expert spends at least two hours each day stretching!

Don't exercise for at least 90 minutes after eating. Digestion and exercise do not go hand in hand. Vigorous exercise will especially upset the early stages of digestion.

Replacing the body's tremendous loss of water due to sweating should follow exercise. This is the best opportunity we have to completely hydrate and purge the body with an abundance of water. If you exercise in a health facility, make sure the water you drink is filtered and does not contain chlorine.

Positive Mental & Spiritual Attitude

"The strength of a man consists in finding out the way God is going, and going that way."

~ Henry Ward Beecher

Maintaining a positive Mental and Spiritual Attitude throughout your life is not as difficult as it may sound. When the mind is confident and rooted in principle and faith, the health of the body will eagerly follow. Like many things, it becomes easy when you make it a habit. We must remember always that the bottom of every valley is the beginning of the next peak to be climbed. But without a positive outlook, Great Health is impossible. Let exercise, the food you eat, and water you drink become a meaningful and integral part of your life, acts of worship if you will. The body is the first temple of God and we must honor it by conditioning it and putting the right foods in to it.

Martial arts preach positive thinking as a central component of their systems because they know that the hand cannot break the board until the mind is convinced that it can. The same is true with health. If the mind doesn't believe it is healthy, the body will be dragged down with it.

Conclusions . . .

One should eat to live, not live to eat. – Molière

There is a subtle yet unmistakable change in thinking about *preventative health* and it is happening worldwide. People are beginning to realize the importance of taking preventative measures to stay in good health such as keeping their bodies alkaline, drinking plenty of water and eating properly. Once a person's body pH becomes unbalanced and overly acid, a plethora of health problems will surely follow, one leading to the next in a cascading effect. We must KNOW which kinds of foods we must eat to remain balanced, renewed and healthy.

Reversing the aging process starts by consuming the water and foods that lead to life. The common sense approach to Great Health, *Spirulina*, *Chlorella*, fresh fruits and vegetables and plenty of *Ionized Water* will bring about an unmistakably positive difference in your health and your life.

Appendix 1
Spirulina, Chlorella and Water Dosages

When and How Much to Take

Chlorella: A maintenance dosage of *Chlorella* is about 3 – 5 grams per day. Although you will not see significant changes taking such a small amount of whole food, your body will be getting a broad array of nutrients unlike it has seen before. Since *Chlorella* is a detoxifying whole food, not a concentrate or extract, a person can eat as much as they desire without any fear of it becoming potentially toxic in any way.

Chlorella is best taken before a meal with probiotics, our friendly bacteria (*Acidophilus* and *Bifidus*). *Chlorella* causes probiotics to multiply at four times the rate of normal.

Maintenance Dosage: 3 – 5 grams/day
Significant Part of the Diet: 6 – 10 grams/day
Immune System Builder: 11 – 14 grams/day
Primary Source of Protein: 12 – 19 grams/day
Healing Purposes & Heavy Metal Detoxification: 20 – 30+ grams/day
Best before a meal to aid with digestion or before a work out.

Spirulina: A maintenance dosage of *Spirulina* is 3 -- 5 grams per day. Although their nutritional profile may appear to be quite similar, *Spirulina* and *Chlorella* are completely different foods.

Spirulina is great before a physical workout. I take 5 – 6 grams religiously before any kind of physical training. Stamina, endurance and recovery are significantly improved with *Spirulina*. After a strenuous workout where the body is pushed to its limits, an additional 10 – 20 grams should be taken during the following 24 hours to rebuild the body and muscle tissue that has been torn down.

Spirulina should also be taken 15 – 30 minutes before a meal to help prepare the stomach for proper digestion since it also helps accelerate the reproductive rate of probiotics.

Maintenance Dosage: 3 – 5 grams/day
Significant Part of the Diet: 6 – 10 grams/day
Immune System Builder: 11 – 14 grams/day
Primary Source of Protein: 12 – 19 grams/day

Healing Purposes: 20 – 25+ grams/day

Water: Water should be consumed each day throughout the day except 30 minutes before, during and at least 30 – 90 minutes after each meal to allow for proper digestion. If you consume water with your meal, it will wash away the probiotics, digestive enzymes and hydrochloric acid that are necessary for proper digestion. You will essentially dilute the entire digestive process by not allowing these crucial digestive bacteria, enzymes and acids to work on the food you consume.

I load up on water 30 minutes before I eat. 45 minutes after you eat, slowly begin to re-hydrate yourself over the next 1 – 2 hours. The digestive process is water intensive and requires an enormous amount of replacement water for the body to remain properly hydrated. Health begins with proper hydration of the body!

Upon waking in the morning, the first order of business should be to re-hydrate the body with 16 – 32 oz. of water.

Consuming half your weight in ounces each day is the bare minimum requirement for water consumption. A 150 lb person would need a minimum of 75 ounces, although I would recommend closer to a gallon each day.

I drink between 1.5 and 2.0 gallons of water per day. Water rocks in the world of Great Health. There's nothing better for our health!

There is no doubt that Chlorella is a food for all generations that will solve many of our health and hunger problems in the coming years.

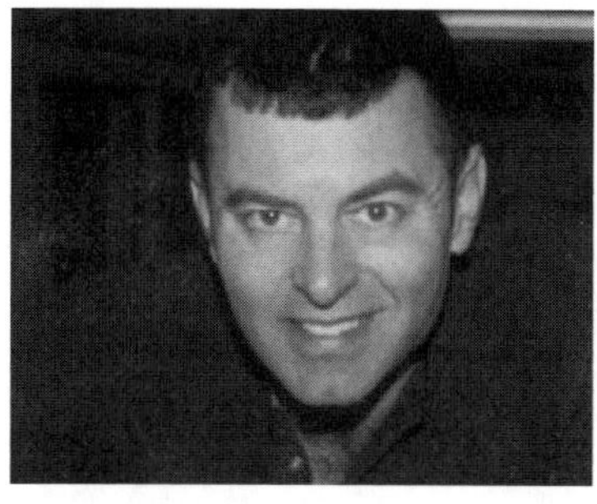

About the Author

Robert F. McCauley, Jr. was raised in Lansing, Michigan, attended Michigan State University (BA, 1980 in Journalism) and worked for several years in New York City at the prestigious law firm of Debevoise & Plimpton. He has traveled extensively, both domestically and abroad, visiting over 32 countries, including India, Korea, France and Israel where he spent significant time. He published Confessions of a Body Builder: Rejuvenating the Body with Spirulina, Chlorella, Raw Foods and Ionized Water in 2000.

From 2002-2004 he hosted a radio Program called **Achieving Great Health**, which was heard by thousands of people each day. It was the first health radio program of its kind, one that promoted natural health in every way and how the body is capable of healing itself of any disease. His guests on the show have included, Peter Ragnar, Dr. Gabriel Cousens, Viktoras Kulvinskas, Dr. Udo Erasmus, Dr. F. Batmangalij, David Wolfe, Jack Lalane, Patricia Bragg and many others in the Raw Food and Natural Hygiene movement. Robert also gives frequent lectures and offers seminars on his natural health protocol.

With the help of his father, Dr. Robert F. McCauley, Sr.[48] (Doctorate; Environmental Engineering, 1953) they started Spartan Water Company in 1992, which sold vended water machines in supermarkets. Robert founded Spartan Enterprises, Inc. in 1993 and began bottling Michigan's best artesian water under the label Michigan Mineral - *Premium Natural Water*, which was sold throughout the Lansing and Detroit areas.

He founded the Watershed, Lansing's first bottled-water store, in 1995. The Watershed is the North American importer of Jupiter Water Ionizers, *Dong Yang Science,* Seoul, Korea. It is also the North American importer of *Chlorella* produced by the Taiwan Chlorella Manufacturing Co. which is the world's largest *Chlorella Pyrenoidosa* producer. It is sold under the name of Watershed Chlorella.

He is a 3rd Degree Black Belt and registered instructor of *Songahm Taekwondo*. He stays young by running, (18:35 - 5 Kilometer race) and following his rules for Great Health laid out in this book. He also enjoys wall and rock climbing.

Index

My Photos

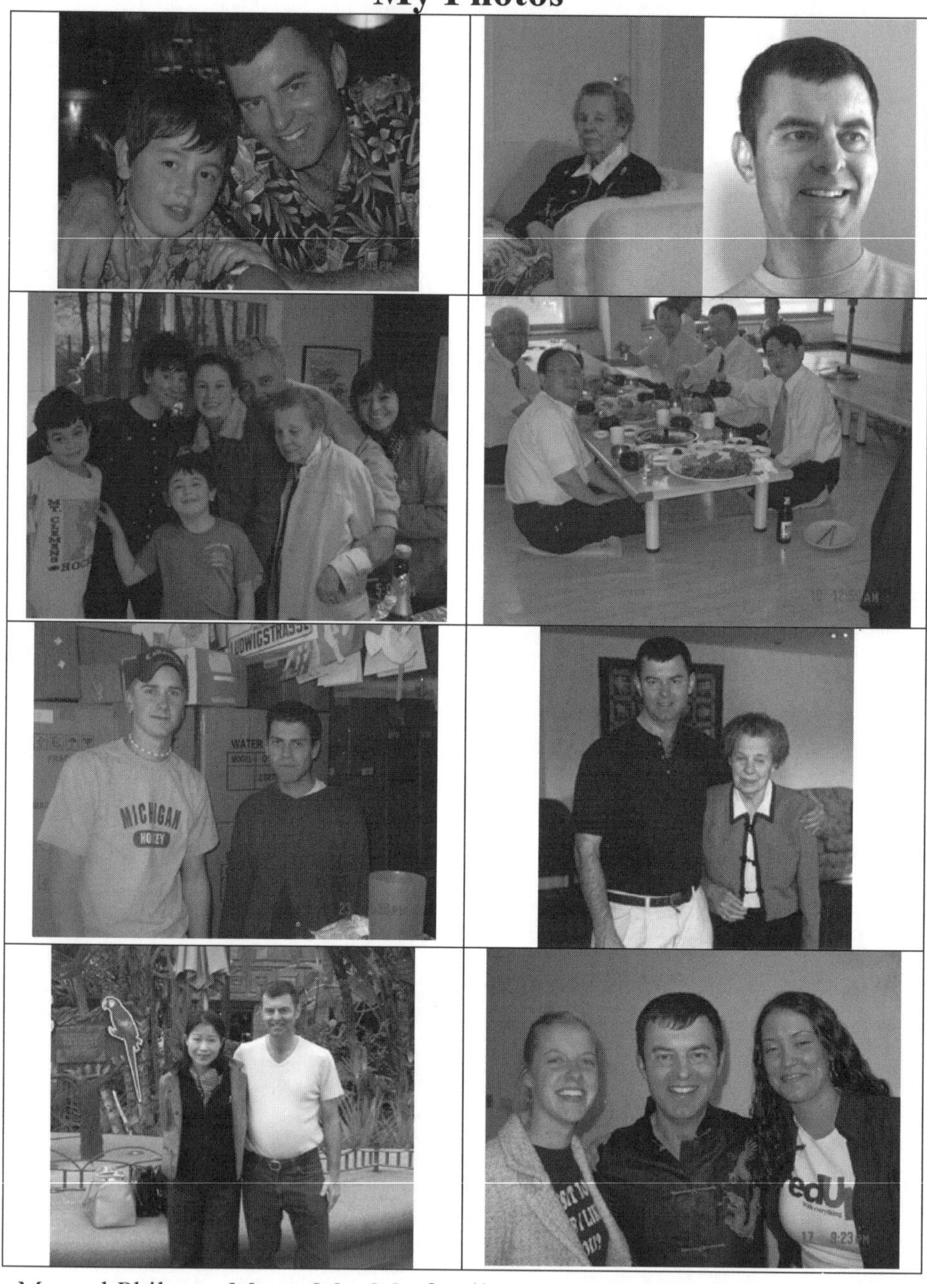

Me and Phil; my Mom; Me; My family; Dong Yang Science Gang, Seoul, Korea 2004; Ryan and Myron; Me and Rose; Me and Ying, Anaheim, CA 2004; Meghan, Me and Patti.

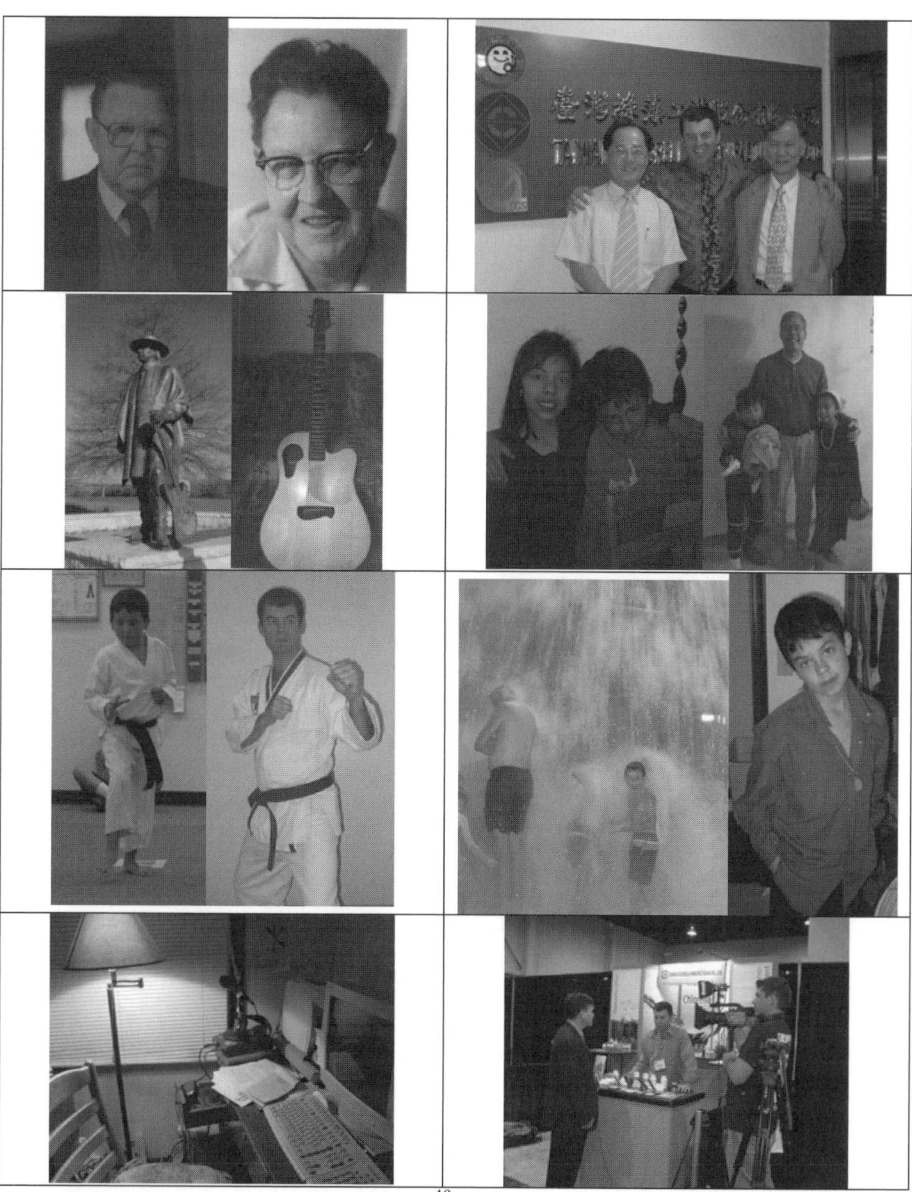

My father, Robert F. McCauley, Sr.[49] (both photos); Mr. Tseng, myself and Mr. Yeh of Taiwan Chlorella Manf. Co., Stevie Ray Vaughn Statue; one of my guitars; Hanna and Phillip, Phillip, Nathan and Hanna; Phillip – Black Belt Testing; Ready Stance; Dan, Me, Phil getting drenched; Dan; My study/Radio Broadcasting Station for Achieving Great Health Radio Program 2003- 2004; Me being interviewed on Chlorella at The Natural Products Expo.

Endnotes

[1] Your Body's many Cries for Water, F. Batmanghelidj, M.D. p. 5

[2] Ibid., p. 25.

[3] Ibid., p. 71.

[4] Ibid., p. 15.

[5] Ibid., p. 6.

[6] Why Purified Water is Bad For You, by Zoltan P. Rona MD, MSc.

[7] Your Body's many Cries for Water, F. Batmanghelidj, M.D. p. 3.

[8] Immanuel Kant, *Philosopher*

[9] Your Body's many Cries for Water, F. Batmanghelidj, M.D. p. 18

[10] Ionized Water Explained, Dr. Hidemitsu Hayashi, Director, The Water Institute, Tokyo, Japan.

[11] Ibid.

[12] Ibid.

[13] Ibid.

[14] Ibid.

[15] Ibid.

[16] Alkalize or Die, by Dr. T. Baroody, p. 18.

[17] Ionized Water Explained, Dr. Hidemitsu Hayashi, Director, The Water Institute, Tokyo, Japan

[18] Alkalize or Die, by Dr. T. Baroody, , p. 20

[19] Acid & Alkaline, by Herman Aihara.

[20] Bone, Acid, and Osteoporosis, The New England Journal of Medicine, June 23, 1994. Vol. 330, No. 25. Editorial.

[21] Food Enzymes for Health and Longevity, by Dr. Edward Howell, p.121.

[22] Young Again! How to Reverse the Aging Process, by John Thomas, p. 107.

---

[23] *Chlorella*, Jewel of the Far East, by Dr Bernard Jensen, D.O., Ph.D, 1978.

[24] *Chlorella*, Special Edition of Health World Magazine 1989

[25] Ibid.

[26] *Chlorella* - Natural Medicinal Algae, by Dr David Steenblock, B.S., M.Sc., D.O.

[27] *Chlorella*, Jewel of the Far East, by Dr Bernard Jensen, D.O., Ph.D, 1978.

[28] *Chlorella* - The sun-powered supernutrient and its beneficial properties, by Michael Rosenbaum, M.D.

[29] *Chlorella* - The sun-powered supernutrient and its beneficial properties, by William H. Lee, R.Ph, ., Ph.D. and Michael Rosenbaum, M.D..

[30] Dr Liang-Pin Lin, National Taiwan University. 1982.

[31] *Chlorella*, Jewel of the Far East, by Dr Bernard Jensen, D.O., Ph.D.

[32] Ibid.

[33] Ibid.

[34] *Chlorella* - Natural Medicinal Algae, by Dr David Steenblock, B.S., ,D.O.

[35] *Chlorella* - The sun-powered supernutrient and its beneficial properties, by William H. Lee, R.Ph., Ph.D. and Michael Rosenbaum, M.D.

[36] *Chlorella*, Jewel of the Far East, by Dr Bernard Jensen, D.O., Ph.D, 1978.

[37] Ibid.

[38] *Chlorella* - The sun-powered supernutrient and its beneficial properties, by William H. Lee, R.Ph., Ph.D. and Michael Rosenbaum, M.D.

[39] *Chlorella* - Natural Medicinal Algae, by Dr David Steenblock, B.S., M.Sc., DO.

[40] *Chlorella*, Jewel of the Far East, by Dr Bernard Jensen, D.O., Ph.D, 1978

[41] Ibid., p. 18

[42] *Chlorella* - The sun-powered supernutrient and its beneficial properties, by William H. Lee, R.Ph., Ph.D. and Michael Rosenbaum, M.D. p. 30

[43] *Chlorella* - Natural Medicinal Algae, by Dr David Steenblock,B.S.,M.Sc.,D.O. p 33.

[44] *Spirulina*, Nature's Superfood., J. Wolf 1992.

[46] Dr. Zimmerman, Ph.D. *President -- Bio-electric-Magnetics Institute*

[47] Conquering Pain. The Air of Healing with BioMagnetism, by Peter Kulish, p. 12

[48] Dr. Robert F. McCauley, Sr., was born and raised in the southwestern United States, Texas and New Mexico. Dr. McCauley served in W.W.II as a Lieutenant Colonel in North Africa and Central Asia. He received his masters' degree from Michigan State University in 1951 and his Ph.D. from the Massachusetts Institute of Technology (MIT) in 1953 for the study of removing radioactive strontium from water. He earned his doctorate in Environmental Engineering in less than 2 years, one of the shortest doctoral studies in the history from MIT. He taught civil, sanitary and environmental engineering at Michigan State University for 20 years before retiring to run Wolverine Engineers & Surveyors of Mason Michigan for 17 years. With his partner they transformed the company into one of most respected and well known engineering firms in mid-Michigan. Dr. McCauley is credited with the invention and development of calcite coating for water main pipes which keep them from rusting. In 1992, he started Spartan Water Company, which provides vended water in supermarkets and was the precursor to Spartan Enterprises and The Watershed Wellness Center.

Published by:
The Watershed Wellness Center
6439 W. Saginaw Hwy.
Lansing, MI 48917
517-886-0440
www.watershed.net